Praise for

THE SCIENCE OF
or Is Gwyneth Paltrow Wr

Winner of the 2015 Science i   y Book Award

"Health and science expert [Timothy Caulfield] debunks the most powerful and persuasive messages being spread by celebrities when it comes to our health and well-being: what works, what doesn't, what is worth our time and money, and what isn't. A fun and informative read."
—*CBC Books*

"[Caulfield] thinks with an academic's rigor and precision and knows the health maintenance territory inside out." —*The New York Times*

"An exhaustively researched, hilarious take on how celebrity culture influences everyday life, from ill-fated attempts to make it big on reality TV to celebrity-endorsed diets and beauty regimens." —*Maclean's*

"An intelligent mix of research and pop culture, Caulfield's analysis of celebrity trends gets to the heart of America's obsession with the fame monster." —*Kirkus Reviews*

"Caulfield's cure for the mess we're in is this lucid and well-researched compendium of the best-available science about diet, fitness, genetics, pharmaceuticals and alternative medicine. . . . A compelling and timely argument for science and a reminder that science is an iterative process, breakthroughs are rare, and there are no magical cures for everything." —Julia Belluz, *The National Post*

"[Caulfield] is dead on about the idea that fame oddly confers a sense of authority about nutrition and fitness. . . . Ambitious . . . he does a good job of taking down the phonies." —*Quill & Quire*

ALSO BY TIMOTHY CAULFIELD

Relax, Dammit!
The Vaccination Picture
The Cure for Everything!

THE SCIENCE OF
CELEBRITY

...or, Is Gwyneth Paltrow Wrong About Everything?

TIMOTHY CAULFIELD

PENGUIN

an imprint of Penguin Canada, a division of Penguin Random House Canada Limited

Penguin Canada
320 Front Street West, Suite 1400, Toronto, Ontario M5V 3B6, Canada

Originally published in hardcover by Viking Canada,
a division of Penguin Random House Canada Limited, in 2015,
and in paperback by Penguin Canada, a division of
Penguin Random House Canada Limited, in 2016, under the title
Is Gwyneth Paltrow Wrong About Everything?: When Celebrity Culture and Science Clash.

Published in this edition, 2020

1 2 3 4 5 6 7 8 9 10

Copyright © 2015 Timothy Caulfield

Library and Archives Canada Cataloguing in Publication

Title: The science of celebrity . . . or is Gwyneth Paltrow wrong about everything? / Timothy Caulfield.
Other titles: Is Gwyneth Paltrow wrong about everything?
Names: Caulfield, Timothy A., 1963- author.
Description: Previously published by Viking Canada under title: Is Gwyneth Paltrow wrong about
everything?: when celebrity culture and science clash. | Includes bibliographical references and index.
Identifiers: Canadiana 20190204893 | ISBN 9780735239777 (softcover)
Subjects: LCSH: Fame—Social aspects. | LCSH: Celebrities—Health and hygiene. | LCSH: Quacks and
quackery. | LCSH: Science. | LCSH: Disinformation. | LCSH: Health products. | LCSH: Popular culture.
Classification: LCC BJ1470.5 .C39 2020 | DDC 306.4—dc23

Cover design: Andrew Roberts
Cover images: Larry Washburn / fStop / Offset.com

Printed and bound in Canada

www.penguinrandomhouse.ca

For the superstars in my life,
Adam, Alison, Jane, Michael and Joanne

CONTENTS

ARE CELEBRITIES MORE WRONG THAN EVER?

I love coffee. I will happily pay an absurd amount for an espresso served by a struggling artist in a hipster café. If desperate for a hit of caffeine, I will buy the cheap stuff from a rundown gas station—even if it has been sitting in a pot stained brown with a decade's worth of residue. But under no circumstances will I pay $135 for a coffee enema.

Gwyneth Paltrow's wellness company Goop markets a product—appropriately, if unimaginatively, called the Implant O'Rama—that is described as an at-home coffee enema system. (Basically, it's a jug with a rubber hose attached to it.) It is part of Goop's recommended "deep detoxification" package—because, apparently, deep detoxification requires a coffee injection into the lower intestine.

It is easy to mock this kind of nonsense and dismiss it as quackery aimed at the misguided and gullible few. But the sale and embrace of this kind of absurd, science-free and potentially harmful product—bowel perforation, abdominal pain, damaged gut microbiome, loss of ability to feel shame, are some of the possible outcomes—has allowed Paltrow's company to grow into a brand worth more than $250 million. And Gwyneth's Goop-y goods are just the tip of a very large and growing pseudoscience-filled iceberg. In the past few years, the wellness industry has ballooned into a market worth more than $4 trillion globally. A significant portion of this money is being spent on products and procedures—like the Implant O'Rama—that are not supported by evidence or even the deployment of common sense.

This embrace of pseudoscience has led many down a dangerous path. Approximately 40 percent of Americans now believe that cancer can be cured solely through the use of alternative therapies, including enzyme and oxygen therapy, diet, vitamins, and minerals. Almost half of young people—individuals between the ages of eighteen and thirty-seven—believe this to be true. There is no evidence to support this idea. In fact, the use of alternative therapies by cancer patients is associated with a significant decrease in survival rates, and with an increase in the refusal of effective, science-based treatments.

Perhaps even more worrisome, we are witnessing the rejection of the science at the core of some of our greatest public health achievements. Vaccines save between two and three million lives every year, most of those children. There is a vast and robust body of evidence supporting the efficacy and safety of vaccines. Yet an increasing proportion of the population has become "vaccination hesitant," facilitating the return and spread of infectious diseases like measles. According to a 2019 poll, a third of Canadians now believe that the science surrounding routine childhood vaccination isn't clear. Another study found that 28 percent of Canadian parents believe in the existence or possibility of a link between vaccines and autism. In other words, a large portion of the population has a degree of vaccination hesitancy based on a fraudulent and completely debunked study. This harmful myth was started by a physician who was discredited and subsequently lost his licence; his paper was retracted and his claim was shown in numerous studies to have absolutely no foundation.

People are attracted to this kind of misinformation for many reasons. There has been an erosion of trust in key institutions, creating a forum for alternate voices, including those from the celebrity sphere. Not surprisingly, research has confirmed that people who embrace alternative medicine are more likely to have a low level of trust in conventional health care. In addition, many in the public may feel their needs are not being met or that science-informed providers are not taking the health issues of their patients seriously. Those concerns may allow unproven approaches and ideas to appear more attractive.

The sway and reach of social media platforms has also increased substantially over the past few years. As historian Sophia Rosenfeld noted, because the internet facilitates the growth of what is popular rather than what is true, it has helped to give rise to the current "culture of untruth." Research tells us that just being exposed to this churning ocean of falsehoods can have an impact on our beliefs and actions. You don't need to be a hard-core conspiracy theorist to be influenced—if only slightly—by a conspiracy theory, be it about the deployment of fluoride as a mind-control drug or the government withholding access to natural cancer cures. Indeed, studies have found that being exposed to fake news and pseudoscientific concepts can alter our memories such that we begin to believe that the "fake fact" has a reasonably credible source. We didn't hear about the value of the alkaline diet from that dreamy football star Tom Brady; we heard about it from a respected nutrition institution. Or so our memory tells us.

This is precisely why Russian trolls use social media to disseminate inaccurate information about things like genetically modified organisms (GMOs) and vaccination. They know that exposure to nonsensical antiscience headlines, memes, and comment-section tirades can help to generate chaos and stir dissent. And that is exactly what it has done.

But it should not be forgotten that celebrities own social media. It is their domain. As of 2019, twenty-one of the top twenty-five Instagram accounts belong to celebrities. (And five of those are members of the Kardashian clan!) The list of the top Twitter accounts is similarly celeb-heavy. When a celebrity uses one of these platforms to share a bit of pseudoscience about a diet, a waist "training" device, an essential oils supplement, a detox routine (Coffee enemas, anyone?), or, worse, a vaccine's safety, it can cross the radar of hundreds of millions of individuals. In a world where 63 percent of people polled say they don't know how to separate trustworthy journalism from falsehoods, where only 27 percent say they feel confident distinguishing factual news from opinion, and where 90 percent admit to falling for fake news, we should not underestimate the impact of this celebrity noise.

Of course, celebrities also continue to take up significant space in the traditional news media. This coverage can facilitate their role in the legitimization and popularization of unproven therapies. Often this is merely a by-product of celebrity news coverage and not a result of an explicit promotional agenda. "Melissa McCarthy Used CBD Oil at the Oscars 2019 Red Carpet to Prevent High-Heel Foot Pain," a February 2019 headline in *US Weekly* reported. That move by McCarthy was deemed "genius" by the magazine, despite the near-complete lack of evidence to support the claim. But credible science is not required for an idea to gain popular appeal, especially if it can hitch itself to the rocket of celebrity. A Google search of the words "Melissa McCarthy," "CBD," and "Oscars" now yields nearly 150,000 results.

Given the power and cultural dominance of celebrity, it is no surprise that the attainment of fame remains a top career ambition of many, particularly young children and adolescents. But over the past few years, the ways in which youth envision a path to fame has shifted away from the traditional star-making vehicles such as acting, singing, and sports. A 2018 survey of primary school children from the UK found that being a social media star—an influencer—was the most-desired celebrity profession. Another study, done for the fiftieth anniversary of the moon landing, showed that kids were three times more likely to want to be a YouTube star than an astronaut. For American and British children between the ages of eight and twelve, being a YouTuber was the most popular answer, selected by a third of the respondents, to the question "What do you want to be when you grow up?"

There are, no doubt, talented people using social media to gain an audience (heck, Justin Bieber and Shawn Mendes were discovered on YouTube). But many social media "influencers" seek a celebrity that is celebrity distilled to its purest form of celebrity-ness. It is fame built on nothing but fame and the ability to utilize that fame as a tool of influence (usually to obtain yet more fame). This isn't celebrity as a side effect of renowned sports skills, musical talent, or acting chops. This is celebrity created through the incremental accumulation of celebrity. That this hollow form of celebrity is now so revered and desired reminds us that fame and influence were, of course, the point all along. As a society we have begun to shed all the (apparently) unnecessary baggage—talent, dedication, insight, creativity, artistic flair—clogging the path. Fame feeds on fame.

Alas, social media influencers are rewarded for their celebrity-for-being-a-celebrity status. It is predicted that consumer brands will dole out $15 billion in 2022 to influencers as payment for social media endorsements, which often means nothing more than using, wearing, or talking about a product online.

But without a doubt, the most definitive recent example of the continued ascendance and power of celebrity was the election of one to the President of the United States in 2016. The success of the "Influencer-in-Chief" was due, in part, to the now-familiar tools of celebrity culture—playing to an audience with branding, bombast, and a social media–empowered spin. The fact that the Trumps and Paltrows of our world can thrive not only by disregarding science, but by wilfully embracing a strategy of untruth, speaks to the depth of the problem we face. This is the era of misinformation, and celebrities are leading the charge.

As an academic who studies the impact of pop culture, I find it exhausting to try to keep up with the daily flood of bunk. But there are glimmers of good news. First, there is growing recognition of the role that pop culture plays in the dissemination of harmful pseudoscience. When this book first came out in 2015, many told me to relax, that Gwyneth and her ilk are just catering to those looking for fun and a bit of harmless luxury. I don't hear that anymore. Indeed, in 2019 the World Health Organization recognized the spread of misinformation as one of the single biggest threats to public health. There is widespread recognition that this topic matters.

Second, regulators have started to take more aggressive action. In 2018, for example, Gwyneth Paltrow's Goop settled a false advertising lawsuit for making deceptive claims about the products they market on the Goop website—claims, for example, that inserting a jade egg into your vagina could improve sex and balance hormones. In addition, regulators, including the US Federal Drug Administration (FDA), have gone after a number of the best-known celebrity-endorsed bunk health products, including IV vitamin treatments, cryotherapy, and unproven stem cell products and procedures.

Finally, many of the social media platforms have taken active steps to curb the spread of pseudoscience. Both Facebook and Instagram have introduced educational pop-ups that appear whenever someone searches vaccine information. These pop-ups contain information from reliable sources, like the US Centers for Disease Control and Prevention (CDC), and are specifically designed to help counter misinformation. Similarly, Google has decided to ban marketing for unproven and experimental health therapies.

On their own, these regulatory actions are likely to have only a moderate impact on the spread of misinformation. Don't get me wrong—they are both welcomed and needed. But there is just too much bunk coming from too many sources for case-by-case policy responses to dramatically alter the landscape in a sustained manner. People like Gwyneth Paltrow will find ways to market coffee enemas and jade eggs and attract followers and expand their lifestyle brands. If I've learned anything during a career battling celebrity pseudoscience, the best defence against the flood of misinformation is fostering the skills necessary to see through the noise. Celebrities aren't going away. Social media isn't going away. Pop culture will continue to spread pseudo-science. But better critical thinking can inoculate individuals against the misinformation. The goal of this book is to help generate, even if only in a small way, the antibodies necessary to separate the sense from the nonsense—an ability needed more than ever.

Now, I'll have another espresso. In a cup, please.

Timothy Caulfield
October 2019

IDOL DREAMS

Damn, I shouldn't have slept so long, is my first thought when I see the size of the line, which is already the width of a boxcar and the length of an aircraft carrier. It is early in the morning and cold. Many of my line mates have blankets and a diminishing food supply. It is clear they have been here for a very long time.

The people in the line come in three categories: teenager, young adult and parent. The last category is, by far, the smallest. And its members are invariably attached to someone from the first category. This makes me an oddball. As far as I can tell, I am the only solo, middle-aged man. I try to look confident and purposeful, as if I am here for some very specific and important reason, but I am sure I look mostly awkward and out of place.

"What are you doing here?" a young woman asks me through a big friendly smile. She is dressed in an outfit that gives her the appearance of someone who just walked off the set of a Mötley Crüe video, circa 1987.

I want to say, "Making a complete fool of myself," especially since I am in serious need of caffeine and do not feel particularly chatty. Instead I offer an ambiguous, "I'm not really sure."

"What are your goals?" I ask the woman, who goes by the not-uncool moniker Shakespeare Sunday.

"I want to make it. And this seems a good place to start," she replies. "*American Idol* needs a rock star!" All of the people within earshot of this last comment raise their arms and let out a loud "*Wooooooo!*" It is as if this group of strangers had rehearsed the moment, which ended in high-fives and fist bumps.

Ms. Sunday hands me her smartphone and invites me to listen to a recording of her work, which is much better than I expected—though I am not sure what I expected. Before the song finishes, Ms. Sunday (I just can't bring myself to call her Shakespeare) notices a commotion down the line and abruptly ends our exchange. She pushes herself toward the edge of the line, grooming herself as she goes. Ms. Sunday has spotted a TV camera.

A man with a microphone is interviewing people in the line, asking them about their hometown, what makes them special and, of course, if they are the next American Idol. As the camera crew tracks the lineup, a wave of preening and posing moves with it. The criteria for selection as an interviewee seem straight-forward: those selected are attractive and/or there is something distinctive about their appearance. My new friend, Ms. Sunday, is among the chosen. She satisfies both requirements, but mostly the latter.

I am not (at least currently) a singer and I do not have any plans to become one. My voice is terrible. Fortunately, my future does not depend on it. I am a university professor who has spent the last twenty years researching and writing about the health policy implications of things like genetics, stem cell research, obesity, health care reform and personalized medicine. So what the heck am I doing at an *American Idol* audition? Well, I hope to audition! And why do I want to audition? Because I want to learn more about and get as close as I can to the phenomenon of celebrity. And nothing represents celebrity culture better than *American Idol*.

Over the past few decades, celebrity culture's grip on our society has tightened. This is a truism. I don't need to convince anyone that we live in the age of celebrity. Yes, celebrities have been part of the cultural landscape for most of human history. From Alexander the Great to Lord Byron, a fascination with the famous has always been with us. But never has celebrity culture played such a dominant role in so many aspects of our lives. As we will see, it has a measurable influence on individual health care decisions, on the things we do to stay healthy, on how we view ourselves physically, on the material goods we want to possess and on our future career aspirations. Whether we like it or not, celebrity culture has a profound impact on our world, framing how we think about important issues and even influencing how we view our place in the universe. But this is not a book *about* celebrity culture—many interesting and thoughtful treatises already exist on the nature and causes of our obsession with famous people. Rather, in this book I analyze and debunk the messages and promises—implicit and explicit—that flow from the celebrity realm, be they about health, diet, beauty, our ambitions or what is supposed to make us happy.

Many definitions of celebrity culture have been proposed. For this book I am interested in our preoccupation with and the value we attach to celebrity lifestyles and to celebrities themselves—whether in the realm of movies, music or sports—and all the industries and social structures that create and sustain them. Celebrity culture is often blamed for the dumbing down of our social discourse, but less has been said about how it is a source of misinformation. Indeed, celebrity culture has emerged as one of the most significant and influential sources of pseudoscientific baloney. It fills our cultural landscape with notions ranging from those that are patently absurd and widely mocked (such as Simon Cowell's hiring of a psychic "house healer" to exorcise his home of "negative energy") to those that gain substantial social traction and market appeal. The popularity of juicing, cleanses, detox diets, weird exercise routines and a boatload of beauty and anti-aging products and practices can be linked directly to celebrity endorsements. Think, for example, of Katy Perry and Hilary Swank's advocacy on behalf of vitamins, Gwyneth Paltrow's enthusiasm for colon cleanses and a gluten-free diet, Jennifer Aniston's ballyhooed belief in water cures, or just about every celebrity's advice on how to lose weight.

Looking at these health and well-being issues through the lens of celebrity culture may seem frivolous. But we should not underestimate the impact celebrities can have on our preferences and attitudes—which is, of course, why they are so frequently paid millions of dollars by advertisers to move product. Specific examples abound. Angelina Jolie's revelation that genetic testing precipitated her decision to have a preventative mastectomy resulted in an immediate increase in demand for both genetic testing and preventative mastectomies. Similarly, and perhaps more damagingly, images of celebrities smoking—in film, on TV shows and in magazines—are linked to an increase in cigarette consumption. The celebrity trend for using beautifying and rejuvenating vitamin intravenous therapy has reportedly caused a shortage of critical medical supplies. Ill-informed celebrity statements about the alleged risks associated with vaccines (most notably by Jenny McCarthy) have adversely impacted public dialogue on the value of vaccines. And, most disturbingly, reports of celebrity suicides are associated with an increase in suicide in the general public. I could go on and on and on.

It has been suggested that humans are evolutionarily wired to follow and, perhaps, be influenced by people they look up to. Many species, including other primates, carefully watch dominant individuals within their group. Evolutionary psychologists have speculated that this tendency evolved as part of a package of innate predispositions that allow humans to learn from successful role models. The process happens unconsciously. While this propensity may have helped prehistoric hunter-gatherers to acquire useful bits of knowledge and skill, in the context of modern society, following Gwyneth Paltrow's health advice or coveting Kim Kardashian's life provides little benefit. In fact, in the pages that follow I will argue that celebrity culture has emerged as one of our society's most pernicious forces, contributing to, among other things, poor health decisions, wasted investments in useless beauty and fitness products, a decreased understanding of how science works, and increased dissatisfaction with our appearance and, perhaps, our lives.

Of course, the impact of celebrity culture reaches well beyond the areas of health and beauty. Increasingly, becoming a celebrity or obtaining a celebrity lifestyle is viewed as a reasonable and obtainable life goal. Even President Obama has commented on the trend. In a 2013 interview he suggested that the constant exposure to "the lifestyles of the rich and famous" has caused "a shift in culture." In the past, "kids weren't monitoring every day what Kim Kardashian was wearing, or where Kanye West was going on vacation, and thinking that somehow that was the mark of success," President Obama said. These comments are both unusual (how many times has the leader of the free world taken time to speculate about the social impact of a reality TV star?) and correct.

As we will see in the chapters to follow, ample evidence supports Obama's observations. Survey research from the United States has revealed that becoming famous is now viewed as a key part of the American Dream. And numerous studies have found that becoming a celebrity—or gaining success in a celebrity-oriented profession such as singing, acting or sports—has emerged as the primary aspiration of a substantial segment of the population. Social media has played a significant role in this development, by bringing celebrities closer to the public and multiplying the opportunities to make social comparisons. The celebrity life seems real, awesome and accessible. One recent study, published in 2013, found that social media interactions with celebrities, particularly through Twitter, allow fans to feel that they have an "authentic" relationship with their idols. They have the sense, rightly or not, that the interactions are real, which in turn leads them to become more "involved and invested in celebrities' lives."

The central goal of this book is simple: to get to the truth about the claims that flow from celebrity culture, be they about the diets that purport to make us thin, the anti-aging products that will keep us forever youthful and wrinkle free, or the actions that we are told we should take, like auditioning for *American Idol*, to propel us into the realm of celebrity. I seek to separate sense from nonsense and provide useable and evidence-informed advice about the strategies that actually work and those that are a complete waste of money and time. I look at everything from vitamins and organic food to gluten-free diets and the chance of making it big as an actor, musician or professional athlete. I also explore the impact of celebrity culture on things like body image, the use of cosmetic surgery and unhealthy behaviors, such as smoking and sunbathing. I examine what it is like to be a celebrity, as well as the social and biological forces that seem to compel many of us to "reach for the stars."

To this end I have deployed a range of traditional scholarly methods, including analyzing the best-available scientific data and interviewing renowned academic and clinical experts. But I have also tried to gain an understanding of various aspects of the celebrity universe and its social impact by interacting with actors, musicians and even porn stars. To put my research in context, I tried celebrity-recommended beauty routines and diets. I signed on with a modeling agency and went to a modeling competition in New York. And I have tried to immerse myself in the celebrity-oriented media. For example, I followed celebrity Twitter feeds, read gossip blogs and forced myself to read every issue— cover to cover—of the world's most popular celebrity-oriented publication, *People* magazine, for an entire year.

The book is organized into three sections, one focusing on health and beauty, one on celebrity ambition, and one on the nature of celebrity life. These sections roughly correspond to the cumulative effect of three celebrity-driven illusions. Part 1 explores the first illusion, which is that celebrity culture embodies a real, achievable and desirable ideal of health and beauty, and confers on celebrities the authority to impart health and beauty advice. Part 2 addresses the second illusion, that the status of celebrity can (and should) be achieved by anyone who dreams/ works/believes in him- or herself with sufficient intensity. This is an illusion I witnessed firsthand at the *American Idol* audition and, as we will see, is central to the role celebrity culture plays in our lives. The final illusion, and the subject of Part 3, is that celebrities lead the happiest, most desirable, most fulfilled lives.

A few words about tone: This book is not meant to mock those who enjoy popular culture or follow celebrities. On the contrary, I *love* celebrity culture. I always have. Indeed, my interest in celebrity culture is one reason I wanted to write this book. When I play *Trivial Pursuit*, the only questions I can reliably answer are the ones from the entertainment category. Each award season, without any effort, I somehow become aware of all the nominees for the Golden Globes, the Grammys, and, of course, the Oscars. I even have a vague knowledge of the celebrities in the running for a People's Choice Award. It is as if the names of the nominees are implanted in my brain as I sleep. I probably know more about Pamela Anderson and Gwyneth Paltrow than about Albert Einstein, Albert Camus or, for that matter, Albert my neighbor. So, if you love and follow celebrity culture, this book is for you.

I am also not going to try to deny or minimize the power of celebrity. Being near the very famous does create an odd, unquantifiable electricity. I felt it myself when, in order to get into the swing of things, I attended the Hollywood premiere of the movie *This Is the End*, starring James Franco, Seth Rogen, Jonah Hill and Emma Watson. I don't mean that I was invited to attend the premiere or to interview the stars. No, I stood outside the theater with hordes of screaming fans waiting for the stars to be delivered in big black limos. At first, I tried to fool myself into believing that I was there as an academic, an impartial observer. I was Jane Goodall in the Hollywood jungle. But as each limo pulled up I got progressively more into it, standing on my tippy toes to see who would emerge from the vehicle.

"Is that James?" I asked no one in particular. It was not. I sighed along with my neighbors. "Oh! It's nobody!"

We all hoped the stars would come to our corner of the line. So we would yell things like "Emma! Emma! Over here!" It didn't work. Pencil-thin Emma Watson waved in our direction but did not stop. But normal-size Seth Rogen did. Indeed, I swear that Seth and I had a moment, locking eyes in a kind of friendly, if silent, Canadian-to-Canadian exchange.

"Seth seems like a nice guy," I said to the guy standing next to me. How the hell would I know that? And why did I want to tell a stranger?

So it's true: celebrities have the capacity to cast a spell on us all. Celebrity culture really is, as the research tells us, a tremendously powerful force. Given this reality, this book is also relevant for those of you who hate celebrity culture—and I know you are out there because I heard from many of you while I was writing about it. If you are looking for further reason to be skeptical of celebrity culture and its impact on our society, the pages that follow will provide you with an abundance of science-informed ammunition.

Shows like *American Idol* leverage this fascination with celebrities and our desire to reap the rewards of celebrity status. Indeed, the promise of becoming a celebrity is the unspoken reward for participating on the show. Hence, my decision to start our journey at an *American Idol* audition.

The massive line of wannabes moves much faster than I expect. *American Idol* is an efficient machine, processing participants like a factory farm processes chickens. Today is only the registration phase. If I satisfy some basic criteria, I will get a wristband that allows me to audition tomorrow morning.

The rules state that I must be an American citizen. Check. A person must not have done well on a previous *American Idol* season. Check. I must not have a current recording contract. Check. I must not have a close personal or family relationship with the company that owns *American Idol*. Check. And I must be between the ages of 15 and 28. Okay, this last requirement could prove to be a challenge.

Still, I have taken this audition seriously. If given the opportunity, I intend to sing "Lost in the Supermarket," by The Clash. Over the past few weeks I have rehearsed a slightly jazzy version of the song in front of my kids, who invariably give me severe Simon Cowell-ish feedback. "Terrible." "Out of tune." "What key was that?" But despite their harsh reviews, I feel that I've prepared a unique and only marginally embarrassing audition piece. I am ready for my chance!

All of the *American Idol* employees wear pale-blue T-shirts embossed with the show's logo and headsets attached to walkie-talkie devices. One of them escorts me to a table where a woman will decide if I can move on to the next phase of the competition. The woman, who is young enough to be a contestant, looks me up and down and I can tell by her you-have-got-to-be-kidding smile and the tilt of her head that her decision has been made. But before she can announce her verdict I launch into a plea.

"Look, I know I am a bit too old," I say quickly.

She grimaces. "A bit?"

"But I really want to do this and I've got a great song prepared!"

Seeing that I am getting nowhere and fearing that I am going to be tossed out, I relent and tell her about my book project. To my surprise, she seems intrigued. After I make my case to the on-site producer, the *Idol* team agrees to let me come back tomorrow. I can't audition, but I can hang with the contestants. Good enough. My jazzy punk styling will need to wait for another day.

I arrive back at the *American Idol* auditions the next morning just as the contestants are gathering under a TV camera attached to the end of a massive boom. The camera swings over the crowd, generating screams and the waving of signs informing the world that the holder has "Got It" and we should "Look No Further," or, of course, that he or she is the "Next American Idol." The scene is repeated again and again as an *Idol* employee with a megaphone calls for more enthusiasm with each pass of the camera.

Currently in its thirteenth season, *American Idol* has developed into a true cultural phenomenon. Tens of thousands of individuals have auditioned for the show. From 2003 to 2011 it was the highest rated show on TV. It is, quite simply, the most popular show of the last decade. Some episodes have attracted nearly forty million viewers. While it has lost momentum over the past few seasons, in 2013 it was still ranked as the seventh most watched regularly scheduled program on TV. And its influence has led to the introduction of other reach-for-the-stars-and-become-a-celebrity shows, such as *America's Got Talent, The*

X Factor, *The Voice* and *So You Think You Can Dance*.

It is no surprise, then, that so many view *Idol* as a vehicle they can ride to superstardom. As I mingle and chat with the contestants, I hear this theme again and again. "Singing is everything," one teenage girl tells me. She is standing alone at the edge of the crowd, wearing a baggie hoodie and jeans, her long hair obscuring much of her face. She views the show as her best chance at fame and fortune because, as she explains, she has "never had any money." As a child she was abused, so when she becomes a star (she tells this in a matter-of-fact tone that suggests she is certain this will happen) she intends to "help the less fortunate." A weak "good luck" is all I can muster in the face of her puzzling optimism.

I chat with many contestants who have been to multiple auditions. One girl with bright-red hair has auditioned five times, never making it past the first round. "Just nerves," she explains. Another, a fifteen-year-old who informs me that "this is her dream" and "something she has wanted her whole life," just finished competing on the rival TV show, *The X Factor*.

While a few people say their expectations are modest, and are auditioning merely for the experience, the vast majority seem to be swinging for the fences. Big-time fame is the goal. They tell me that you must "reach for the stars" and "hold on to your dreams" and "continue to believe" and that singing is "the number-one priority in life."

Then a strange thing happens. I look up from my notepad and find a small crowd gathering around me—a tight semicircle of smiling contestants eager to be interviewed. Some are throwing my way bits of biographical information about their age, their experience and their multiple talents. It occurs to me that they think I am from a reputable newspaper or magazine, but my explanation that I am working on a book project does little to dampen the enthusiasm. Everyone wants to be interviewed. They want exposure. Just when I start to worry that my little scrum might get out of hand I am saved by none other than Ryan Seacrest.

"Who is ready to change their life today?" Seacrest screams. "Is the next American Idol here?" Everyone goes berserk.

Seacrest moves through the crowd, a camera crew recording his genial interactions with the contestants. He comes closer and closer to my position. And just when it seems possible that he is going to back into me, I make a fatal mistake. I take out my phone and snap a few pictures. Who can blame me? It's Ryan Seacrest! He is so close I could touch his perfectly coiffed hair.

A headset-wearing *Idol* employee taps me on the shoulder. "Excuse me," she says, "but you don't belong here."

PART I

THE ILLUSION OF CELEBRITY AUTHORITY

CHAPTER 1

DIETING, GWYNETH AND MY CLEANSE

Donna Karan and Demi Moore are just two among many celebrities who have raved about the diet regime that just about everyone associates with Gwyneth Paltrow. Indeed, if celebrity endorsements were proof of a product's effectiveness, the Clean Cleanse that Gwyneth is always talking about would be beyond criticism. So it seems to me that the obvious place to start my investigation into the cleanse is in London, home of Gwyneth's booming e-commerce company, Goop. I figure I will ask the employees of Goop about the Gwyneth-inspired cleanse experience before I try it myself. Gwyneth often writes about it in her frequent Goop blogs. She has said "this thing is amazing" and that it "worked wonders" and that it made her feel "pure and happy and much lighter." She has also noted that it is something that she does with the whole "Goop team."

I'd love to feel pure, happy and lighter. Okay, I'm not sure what that would feel like, but it sounds better than I usually feel. Who wouldn't want to feel like that? Given the warm and friendly vibe on the Goop website—it was, after all, to quote the website, "created to celebrate all life's positives"—I am expecting a warm and happy vibe at Goop HQ.

I am mistaken. Apparently, I am not one of life's positives.

I ring the buzzer to request entry to the second-floor office. No response. I try again, and then again. Still no response. I implement Plan B. A courier is buzzed up and I do the classic foot-in-the-door move. I feel like Jason Bourne.

I confidently walk up to the Goop receptionist and give her a friendly hello. She does not say "May I help you?" or even "Do you have an appointment?" Instead I get a blank, Goopless stare. Undaunted, I ask to see someone about the cleanse, trying my best to give the impression that I am here for a prearranged meeting. She looks at me as if I am a homeless man asking for spare change. In other words, she doesn't look at me. She picks up the phone—still not a word to me—to tell someone about my presence in the office. Then I wait. And wait. Just when I start to fear a Goop security guard will appear, doubtless wearing a tasteful, Stella McCartney–inspired ensemble, a young woman approaches me. "You're here to talk about the Clean Cleanse?" she says brightly.

Finally! I think. *This is more like it. My dogged journalistic persistence has paid off.* "That's right," I say. "I'd really like to know more about what actually takes place in the cleanse. I want to get some details about the process and the science behind it."

She smiles. "What a good idea."

This is unfolding precisely as I'd hoped it would. "Thank you," I say. "Who would you suggest I speak with?" I imagine Gwyneth herself now cooperating with my investigation.

"I would say Dhru Purohit," says the charming young lady.

I take out my notebook, expecting her to lead me down the hall to the office of said person. "And where would I find him?"

"Santa Monica, I believe." Her smile now is accompanied by an arched eyebrow. "Which is where the Clean Program is based.

You know that, right? That they're the company that makes the Clean Cleanse?"

I close my notebook. Jason Bourne did not have to implement Plan B to exit the building.

After a few phone calls and emails about my desire to do the cleanse, Dhru Purohit has a kit sent to my house (the usual price is $425). He also invites me to the Santa Monica office to offer some pre-cleanse advice and to meet the guru himself, Dr. Alejendro Junger.

The building is inconspicuous. It is not the type of structure you would expect for the head office of a wildly successful diet company. The Clean Program has produced several international bestselling books and tens of thousands of Clean Cleanses, which the company website heralds as "the most endorsed, supported and effective cleanse in the world." And yet their offices, just a block off Los Angeles's often-sung-about Santa Monica Boulevard, look like a modest walk-up apartment. *Do they live here?* I wonder as I approach the door. There is no sign announcing the name of the company. Not even a nameplate; just a buzzer.

But if the building is understated, its occupants are not. When it comes to life's positives, the Goop team could learn a thing or two from Dhru Purohit. This guy is fun. He is all energy, enthusiasm and commitment. "Hey, Tim!" Purohit says with a big, welcoming smile as soon as the door swings open. He invites me into the company's modern workspace, which looks more like an open-concept home than a business. No offices, cubicles or desks in sight—just a large kitchen and several comfy-looking sofas and chairs. Purohit tells me he is "a Sherpa of sorts." He's a guy who "enjoys guiding people and communities through the world of holistic healing and spiritual living." And he believes in the cleanse product the way Napoleon believed in the flexible use of artillery. It may not be easy to implement, but it can change the world.

Dr. Junger is scheduled to arrive in a few minutes, so I take the time to ask Purohit about what I view as the biggest challenge associated with the cleanse: no coffee. "I am a coffee addict," I tell him. "I love coffee. I cannot stress this enough. It is central to my very existence. Are you sure I must give it up?"

"You must give your adrenals a rest," he explains. "And you must remove the dependency. The idea that you need coffee to function, long term, stresses your adrenals. Your adrenals are your energy bank account." I will hear the word "adrenal"—which, I assume, is a reference to the hormones secreted by the adrenal glands—approximately nine thousand times during my interactions with the Clean Program teams. *Adrenal glands. Adrenal fatique. Adrenal stress. Adrenal rest.*

Moments later Dr. Junger arrives. I will say this about the man: He projects a relaxed energy. He's got his adrenals in check, obviously. His posture is relaxed, his voice is relaxed and his outfit is relaxed. I am pretty sure he is wearing hand-knitted slipper shoes. I can see why Gwyneth likes hanging with him. I feel more Zen just being in his presence.

Purohit tells Junger about my cleanse plan. "It. Will. Blow. Your. Mind," Junger tells me as he settles into one of the comfy chairs, legs crossed as if he is about to meditate.

Dr. Junger is a physician from Uruguay. He is the inventor of the Clean Cleanse and is often described in the popular press as Gwyneth Paltrow's doctor, though "spiritual leader" would probably be more accurate. Indeed, Gwyneth's bestselling cookbook, *It's All Good*, is dedicated to Dr. Junger, among others, whom she describes as "her good friend." The book contains recipes inspired by Dr. Junger's diet and health philosophy. In the preface, she credits him, and the Clean Cleanse, with curing her of a variety of ailments, including the banishment of an intestinal parasite that went undetected by Gwyneth's conventional physicians, the adjustment of her "sky-high" adrenals and the unclogging of her horribly clogged liver. If you believe Gwyneth, the cleanse reduced her levels of stress and improved her looks. Given all this Gwyneth attention, it is no surprise that Dr. Junger is a bit of a celebrity himself, appearing on shows such as Dr. Oz, where he provides detoxing and cleansing advice.

He explains to me how the cleanse works and why it is so important, making many references to detoxification, our body's energy systems, our body's natural ability to heal, the evils of gluten and, naturally, adrenals. He also compares our world to a dirty fish tank filled with "toxic triggers" such as plastic, pollution and drugs. "The dirty fish tank is, for us, the city. It is unnatural. The more industrialized, the more chemicalized, the more diseases there are." I am not sure that a medieval serf would agree with his analysis, but I get the idea.

At the risk of sounding unconcerned for my fellow Earth-dwellers, I tell him that my biggest concern is whether I can hack it or not. "I'm worried it's going to be too tough," I tell him, my thoughts centered on the coffee ban. "I don't think I can do it."

"Don't declare something you don't know," Dr. Junger says. "Keep an open mind. Go with it. You should be thinking 'I wonder how this is going to transform me?'"

I am three days into my cleanse and my family is not impressed. They are ready to cleanse me from their lives. My sanity is questioned. My company avoided. And my eating habits characterized as revolting. And, to add insult to self-inflicted injury, I am told my breath stinks.

At this stage I do not feel clean or pure or happy. I feel and behave like a miserable bastard. The combination of caffeine withdrawal and hunger pangs has transformed me into a feral beast with a fuse as short as one of Gwyneth's fabulous dresses. (Specifically, I'm thinking of that minimalist number she wore to the opening of her fitness studio in Hollywood. The dress is a Victoria Beckham design, I believe. But the lack of coffee has left me pretty confused, so I can't be sure. Perhaps it was an Alexander Wang.)

You are probably wondering what the cleanse involves. What is the magic formula that will transform me? Here are the basics. For breakfast I suck back a shake made out of a prepackaged powder that looks but does not taste like the chocolate milk mix I loved as a kid. It is neither appetizing nor satisfying. I must use almond or coconut milk because no dairy products are allowed. This concoction is also my evening meal. Every evening. Needless to say, I go to bed hungry. For lunch I can have real food, but the selection is greatly restricted. Apples are okay, but not bananas. Lemons yes, oranges no. No raisins. I can have organic chicken and wild fish, but no beef or pork. No wheat or gluten, naturally. Sugar is verboten (though the fact that many foods have naturally occurring sugar in them is never addressed by the Clean Program team). No eggs. And, sadly, because I really feel like I could use some, no alcohol. I must also consume a variety of supplements, including a boatload of probiotics.

I showed my colleague, Professor Linda McCarger, a renowned clinical nutritionist and metabolism researcher, the ingredients of the Clean Cleanse shake mix and supplements. "Looks like they are simply trying to remove everything often associated with an allergic response. They seem to be working off the gluten-free, allergy-free trend," is her initial reaction to the information sheet provided by the Clean Program. I was curious about some of the specific ingredients in the chocolaty powder; in general, she saw nothing unique in them. "They have components like rice syrup. But there is nothing special about that. It is just not made from wheat ... but it is still a sweetener, used by the body like other syrups. No magic."

This spartan, not-magic existence lasts for twenty-one days. As of my meeting with Linda, I've got seventeen to go. I have serious doubts about whether I can make it. I keep reminding myself that Gwyneth does this on a regular basis. She is tougher than I thought.

Cleansing, driven largely by celebrity endorsements, has become an extraordinarily popular trend. It now involves the sale of special detoxifying juices (currently estimated to be a $5 billion market), cleansing programs (such as the one I am on) and colon cleanses (yep, exactly what it sounds like). There is also a baffling array of books on cleansing and detoxification. Here is a far-from-comprehensive list of just the books that have duration as their primary theme, in descending order of urgency: *The One Month Carb Detox*; *The 4-Week Ultimate Body Detox Plan*; *The 21-Day Sugar Detox*; *The 14-Day Detox Diet*; *The 12-Day Detox Guide*; *The 10-Day Detox Diet*; *The 9-Day Liver Detox Diet*; *The 8-Day Detox Breakthrough*; *The 7-Day Detox Miracle*; *The 6-Day Detox Drop*; *The 5-Day Kidney Detox*; *The 4-Day Detox* (not to be confused with the *Detox 4 Women*); *The 3-Day Green Smoothie Detox*; *The Food Combining 2-Day Detox*; and, for those in a real hurry, *The Fast Track One-Day Detox Diet*.

The concept of cleansing and detoxifying rests on the idea that due to all the toxins in the modern world, and all the crap we eat, our bodies need to be scrubbed clean. By doing this, or so the theory goes, we will promote natural healing, reduce stress (the adrenals thing) and reset (a word often associated with cleanses) our system. Cleanses are also presented as a way to look healthier and lose weight. For example, Katy Perry told the world, again and again, that she went on a three-month cleanse that included vitamins and supplements in preparation for the photo shoot she did for her July 2013 cover of *Vogue*. This was because, as Perry said, she "just wanted to be glowing for that cover."

To be fair, celebrities endorse or are associated with a range of health-related activities, from environmental causes to the support of biomedical research. And many crazy celebrity diets are promoted. But the current cleanse trend provides the perfect opportunity to examine the claims so often associated with extreme celebrity-driven fads. It also provides an opportunity to look at what science tell us about how we should eat and what is really good and bad for us.

CLEANSING AND DETOXIFYING

Let's start with the central idea. Do our bodies need to be detoxified and will cleansing do the trick?

No and no.

Despite the remarkable popularity of the practice, absolutely no evidence supports the idea that we need to detoxify our bodies in the manner suggested by the cleansing industry. The proponents of cleansing often sell the idea by using colorful metaphors that make it all seem so darn logical. The manual for the Clean Cleanse puts it this way: "If you don't take out the trash at your house, it will pile up, attract pests, and quickly become a problem. Having daily bowel movements will help make sure that toxins aren't re-absorbed into your system."

Who wants trash and pests in their colon?

Do not be fooled by these rhetorical games. The idea of detoxing is faulty on so many levels that it borders on the absurd. First, the human body has organs, including the kidneys, liver, skin and colon, that take care of the detoxification process. When you pee, you are detoxifying. Toxins don't build up waiting to be cleansed by supplements and special foods. (And, just in case you are wondering, you don't reabsorb toxins by not having your regular bowel movement. Sigh.) No evidence suggests that we need to assist our detoxifying organs by ingesting specific foods or supplements. As summarized in a 2005 academic article titled "Detox Diets Provide Empty Promises," "These approaches are contrary to scientific consensus and medical evidence and are not consistent with the principle that diets should reflect balance, moderation, and variety."

Second, and more importantly, no evidence suggests that the products and diets sold by the cleansing industry—whether juices, supplements or specific diet regimens—do anything to help clear toxins, parasites or bad karma in a manner beneficial to our health. Not one single scientific study appears to back up the theory behind this massive industry. (Okay, I found *one* study, published in the *Journal of Chiropractic Medicine*, that involved seven individuals and no comparator group. The methods are so poor that I am not sure it qualifies as a study.) The British Broadcasting Corporation (BBC) did a fun and somewhat scientific-ish experiment involving ten "party animal" young adults. Five got a balanced diet that included, in moderation, stuff usually viewed as "toxic triggers" (coffee, chocolate, fries, etc.) and five were put on a detox regimen. After a week they ran a bunch of tests, including testing for antioxidants and kidney and liver function. The result? No difference. The detoxing didn't do anything.

An interesting analysis done by thirty-six young scientists for an independent organization called The Voice of Young Science (where do I send my check?) looked at the science behind fifteen popular detox products. Among other things, they contacted the manufacturers and asked them for evidence. (Alas, the Clean Cleanse was not studied.) What did they find? *No one* was able to provide any solid evidence to support the detox claims. Remember, they asked the people who made the products! You'd think they'd have a bit of real evidence handy. Also, they found that there wasn't even a consistent or comprehensive definition of what is meant by "detox" and, to quote the study, "Many of the claims about how the body works were wrong and some were even dangerous." As a result, the thirty-six young scientists conclude: "'detox' as used in product marketing is a myth."

The reality is that a good study on the efficacy of cleanses would, from a methodological perspective, be fairly complicated, requiring large, long-term trials that have individuals on a variety of different cleansing programs and diets. And ideally, the research method would also elucidate the mechanism of action. So we need to take care not to read too much into experiments such as the one conducted by the BBC. But you simply can't assert, as so many detox sales pitches do, that certain foods magically flush evil toxins out of the system. What toxins? Where do they reside? How do the foods, supplements, vitamins, etc., work?

Many cleanse and detox programs also refer to the idea of creating a healthy gut. Again, this is a big theme for Gwyneth and Dr. Junger. Interesting studies have shown how gut bacteria affect a range of health topics, from psychological well-being to obesity. However, this science, which is still in its early stages, gives cause for caution in the context of cleanses. Before we fiddle with our feces, so to speak, we should recognize that the bacteria that live in our gut play a complex and important role in our health. At the current time, no one (seriously, *no one*) knows if and how we can adjust our diet to alter the microbes in our gut in a manner that will maximize health.

"Existing research tells us it is very difficult to reset your [gut bacteria]. You can't easily control what goes on. Even if you can change it, it will just go back to exactly where it was before," Karen Madsen tells me. "Gut bacteria is pretty resilient."

Madsen is a professor of gastroenterology and co-director of the University of Alberta's Centre of Excellence for Gastrointestinal Inflammation and Immunity Research. She is intrigued by my cleanse experiment and suggests that I get my gut material—which is, basically, my feces—tested during and after my cleanse. The process of collecting "samples" and bringing them to her lab in a (thankfully) opaque plastic container is not fun. But, as we will see, the results are instructive.

Even the idea that we have toxins floating around our bodies is sketchy. Beyond fuzzy references to our dirty environment, the evils of pesticides and pharmaceuticals (for some reason, supplements are okay), rarely do the advocates of cleanses explain what is meant by "toxins." It is one of those nebulous pseudoscientific terms rolled out by people deliberately avoiding the specificity required for a science-based analysis. It is the modern-day equivalent of "evil spirits." It is vague enough to mean just about anything while retaining the ring of scientific legitimacy. Every common health complaint—low energy, fatigue, amorphous pain, insomnia, anxiety, general malaise, etc.—can be attributed to the existence of toxins. But what, exactly, do the detoxification experts mean? Do they mean the natural poisons that reside in the environment? Do they mean only human-made chemicals? If so, which ones and why? Do they mean junk food? Do they mean all of the above? If so, how are their magical treatments designed to address such vastly different compounds and conditions?

As Joe Schwarcz, director of McGill University's Office·for Science & Society, told me when I asked him to sum up the detox fad, "What really needs to be detoxified is the concept of detox."

I can't resist commenting on Dr. Junger's city-as-a-dirty-fish-tank analogy. The idea that many of us live in toxin-filled, disease-ridden urban bogs is often a core part of the we-must-cleanse narrative. You see it reflected in the images found in Gwyneth's cookbook: Gwyneth sitting in a field in the country. Gwyneth hanging with a friend at a picnic table in the country. Gwyneth riding a red scooter in the country. The whole book has an old-timey country feel. But despite the long-held belief that living in the (allegedly) toxin-free fresh air and wide-open spaces of our rural regions is intrinsically healthy, the available evidence does not support this cliché. While health risks are certainly associated with both urban and rural settings—and, if you had a time machine, hanging out in pre-sewage-system London would not be a health-promoting decision—research has consistently shown that contemporary cities are healthier than rural retreats, particularly if you are lucky enough to reside in the middle to upper socioeconomic strata (where, I am pretty sure, most "detoxifiers" are found). City dwellers, on average, are slimmer, smoke less and are more active. Rural dwellers are, on the other hand, more likely to have health issues such as strokes, diabetes, high blood pressure and some forms of cancer.

A review article published in the *American Journal of Public Health* concluded that "premature mortality (dying before the age of seventy-five) is greater among rural residents than among urban residents." Another, published in 2014, found that "life expectancy was inversely related to levels of rurality." While much of this difference can be attributed to socioeconomic status, this isn't the whole story. A study published in 2013, for example, found that "youth in rural areas had significantly higher mortality rates than their urban counterparts regardless of deprivation levels [i.e., socioeconomic status]." And other studies have found that the urban poor fare better, from a health perspective, than the nonurban poor. Cities have problems too, of course. Some evidence indicates that higher levels of sexually transmitted disease exist in urban areas. Also, a 2011 study from Canada found that people living in rural settings had a lower risk of depression, likely because of a stronger sense of community. But contrary to the claims made by many of the detoxification prophets, cities should not be viewed as dirty disease-causing fish tanks. Indeed, "urbanization appears to be a force for better health," as noted by Christopher Dye, the director of health information at the World Health Organization, in an oft-cited article from the journal *Science*.

Don't get me wrong. I am not a fan of pollution, which cities usually (but not always) have at higher concentrations than other regions. Pollution is not good for our health. Tentative evidence even shows that, for instance, prenatal exposure to a specific pollutant—the by-product of burning fossil fuels, polycyclic aromatic hydrocarbons—can increase the risk of obesity. And I have no objection to the fresh food and active lifestyle so often (erroneously, as it turns out) associated with country life. But no evidence indicates that, in the aggregate, cities are inherently unhealthy. Also, no evidence suggests that living in a city is a reason to cleanse. We urbanites aren't fish in a dirty tank.

So, what were the results from my gut test?

The cleanse had absolutely no impact. The Gwyneth cleanse, which is darned extreme, did not change the makeup of the bacteria in my colon. Remember, fixing or "resetting" your gut is one of the alleged goals of cleansing. Madsen's conclusion regarding the condition of my fecal matter is definitive: "Pretty healthy looking I would say, and the cleanse did nothing at the phylum level! Your microbes appear to be pretty resilient, which is a good thing."

Inexplicably, I feel a small burst of excreta pride, as if Madsen's assessment of the vast community of microorganisms living in my intestine is a tribute to my character. "Why, thank you …"

STRESS, HAPPINESS AND ADRENAL FATIGUE

Many cleanses, including the Clean Cleanse, are also aimed at reducing the emotional and physiological stress caused by a variety of food and environmental toxins. This was a big theme during my discussions with the Clean Program team in Santa Monica. And it is often reported that this is why celebrities go on cleanses: they need to recharge as a result of their hectic celebrity life. Again, this is a point that Gwyneth makes in the preface to *It's All Good*.

So, is there any science to suggest this works?

Some evidence does imply that eating a healthy diet can have a tangible impact on mood. For example, a 2013 study of 281 young adults found that eating fruits and vegetables was associated with a positive emotional state. A similar 2013 study, from Finland, examined the eating habits of more than two thousand individuals and found that a healthy diet, particularly one that emphasizes fruits and vegetables, was protective against depression. Studies have also found that junk food is associated with depression. A 2012 study from Spain followed the eating habits of almost nine thousand individuals and found that "fast-food and commercial baked goods consumption may have a detrimental effect on depression risk." And early-stage research shows that the bacteria in our gut can also have an impact on mood. One small study from UCLA, for example, examined the impact of eating a particular type of yogurt on brain function. The study, which included before and after brain scans, found that the consumption of probiotic yogurt (which, incidentally, I wasn't allowed to eat while on my cleanse!) altered, for the better, how the brain processed information and reacted to negative stimuli.

A school of research looks at stress, as measured by biomarkers such as the level of cortisol (often called the stress hormone) in both blood and urine. Studies have found, for example, that a healthy diet may help to reduce stress and protect against its adverse physiological effects. It is also worth noting, however, that this works in the opposite direction too: high stress causes us to eat poorly. A 2013 study from Belgium, for example, measured the cortisol level of 323 children between the ages of five and ten. The measurements were taken three times a day. It was found that higher levels of cortisol (i.e., more stress) were linked to an unhealthier diet, including the consumption of fatty foods and more snacks. This may be why we reach for comfort food when stressed out.

While much of the food and happiness research is preliminary or marred by methodological limitations (e.g., does eating lots of fruits and vegetables make you happy or do happy people eat lots of fruits and vegetables?), I do believe it is likely that the diet can impact mood and how we handle stress. At a minimum, a healthy diet will make us more resilient and healthier in general, which is, of course, going to help with our emotional well-being.

So, yes, it is possible—in fact, highly probable—that what we put in our mouths can have an impact on our stress level and mood. But not one stitch of evidence suggests that the particular protocols recommended by the various cleanse programs will have this effect, at least not for the reasons offered by their proponents. Indeed, the preliminary status of this research should remind us that any definitive claim of causation—for example, that certain foods or supplements ease stress and alter hormone levels—is premature. At this stage, the research merely suggests that we should strive to eat a healthy, balanced diet. It does not support the idea that some form of extreme diet—and it is fair to categorize most cleanses as extreme—will improve your long-term emotional well-being and your stress levels as measured by biomarkers.

In fact, at least some research suggests that these kinds of diets have the opposite effect, putting our bodies under unnecessary stress. (I certainly felt stressed during my cleanse!) For example, a 2010 study of 121 females found that a diet that greatly restricted calories *increased* blood cortisol levels and the self-reported perception of stress, thereby leading, ironically, to an eventual increase in calorie consumption.

In addition, we need to be cautious in assessing the utility of particular tests as a method for diagnosing an individual's level of stress and well-being. Little or no evidence suggests that tests that reveal "sky-high adrenals," for example, have any bearing on health or well-being. While measuring the hormones cortisol or adrenaline—two of the main adrenal hormones—can be useful if a deficiency or excess is demonstrated (e.g., adrenal insufficiency is a *real*, but relatively rare, ailment, which happens when something is physically wrong with the adrenal glands), measurements must be taken throughout the day and at the appropriate time. A 2010 systematic review, which is a rigorous analysis of all the available evidence, looked at the utility of a range of tests, including measurements for cortisol, for the detection of "burnout," the term often used to describe the state of stress associated with exhaustion, fatigue, loss of energy, etc. After carefully analyzing thirty-one studies, the authors concluded, "No potential biomarkers for burnout were found."

Jacques Romney, a University of Alberta colleague of mine and an associate professor of endocrinology, agrees with this assessment. He told me that while cortisol and adrenaline are indeed relevant to how the body responds to stress, using a result to see "how stressed the body might be" is inappropriate: "Cortisol and adrenaline are part of the body's response to stress. However, these hormones naturally fluctuate throughout the day, so one cannot pick a certain lab value and determine how stressed one is in day-to-day life."

In fact, the whole concept of "adrenal fatigue" (or "adrenal burnout" or "adrenal exhaustion" or whatever you want to call it) is very controversial. The theory is that emotional stress and exposure to certain toxins, such as coffee, exhausts the adrenal glands, resulting in a variety of nebulous symptoms (fatigue, feeling overwhelmed, etc.). It was partly to relieve my adrenals that I was told to get off coffee as part of my cleanse. As Dr. Junger suggests in the book *Clean*, "When caffeine is taken in persistently over a period of time, one can exhaust the adrenal system and not even realize caffeine was the cause."

A lot of conflicting (and scientifically inaccurate) information about this "ailment" can be found floating around the internet. Indeed, it has been called by skeptics an "internet disease," because, to quote a commentary in the *LA Times*, it exists "only in the minds of people who post about [it] on the Internet." It is fair to say that most researchers in the medical and scientific community do not recognize it as a real condition. The endocrinologists I interviewed were blunt in their assessment: adrenal fatigue/exhaustion does not exist and testing for it is likely useless. A statement from the endrocrinologists' professional organization, the Hormone Society, which is the public education arm of the Endocrine Society, is also pretty unequivocal. Specifically, it states, "'Adrenal fatigue' is not a real medical condition. There are no scientific facts to support the theory that long-term mental, emotional, or physical stress drains the adrenal glands and causes many common symptoms." And, just so there is no mistake, they also make the point that "there is no test that can detect adrenal fatigue."

I am not going to take a definitive stand on the concept of adrenal fatigue or the whole idea of testing to see if your "adrenals" are "sky-high." I don't need to. My point is more modest: you should not believe anyone who suggests, either explicitly or implicitly, that an authoritative biological test for life stress exists. And you can confidently reject any assertion to the effect that adrenal fatigue/burnout/stress is a well-established condition. More importantly, given the scientific uncertainty about the nature (or, even, existence) of the problem, don't believe anyone who claims to have a remedy!

WEIGHT LOSS

Let's be honest, the primary reason that people cleanse is not for the benefit of some de-stressing, spiritual, soul-centering purification process. It is for the purpose of weight loss. The main motivation for many of the things we do related to our health, especially dieting, has to do with how we look. And when cleanses are discussed in the popular press, particularly when a celebrity name is invoked, weight loss is almost always the focus. Shape.com, for example, tells us Salma Hayek "credits her slim and sexy shape to the juice cleanses" and that "Beyoncé turned to the Master Cleanse Diet to help her drop a reported 20 pounds in less than two weeks." Similarly, Gwyneth's cleanses are often depicted as the secret to her slim body. A February 2014 article in *People* magazine provides a lighthearted analysis of the effectiveness of the cleanses used by Beyoncé, Kyra Sedgwick, Mindy Kaling and, naturally, Gwyneth. And by effectiveness, *People* means just one thing: weight loss. Not a single word is offered about actual, scientifically derived, evidence in relation to health, but much is said about the number of pounds lost, which ranged from five in twenty-two days to the relatively extreme twelve in fourteen. So, for all the claims made for them, cleanses are little more than an extreme diet. They are a way to lose weight fast. Indeed, back in Santa Monica, Purohit admitted to me that 80 percent of their customers are "interested primarily in weight loss."

How about my own cleanse-induced weight loss? Every morning I get naked and anxiously step on our bathroom scale. Gwyneth, Junger and Purohit will be happy to hear that their cleanse is causing me to lose more than just my dignity. The hard-to-stomach shakes and limited menu options are working their slimming magic. Abracadabra! The weight is disappearing. In my starved state, I can imagine globs of toxins and unhealthy impurities being flushed from my gluten- and coffee-free system.

My morning weigh-in has become the highlight of my day. Like a lab rat getting a hunk of cheese, the weight loss serves as a tangible sign that the cleanse is doing something. As I look down at the number on my bathroom scale, I can hear Dr. Junger's soothing voice remind of how this experience would "transform me." Is this what he meant?

But is cleansing a good weight-loss strategy? You can probably guess the answer. Let's start by reviewing what the evidence tells us about weight loss. It isn't pretty. It is, sigh, nearly impossible to keep weight off. Study after study has found that while people can lose weight, sustained weight loss is the true challenge. Even the studies that are structured like clinical trials—that is, the participants are carefully monitored by health care professionals—have found that the vast majority of people can sustain only modest weight loss, regardless of the type of diet used. (In these studies, successful weight loss is usually defined as keeping off 5 to 10 percent of a person's initial weight—not exactly the beach-ready transformation promised by, to cite one example, the "Bikini Detox Diet.") A well-known study published in 2007 carefully analyzed twenty of the most methodologically sound dieting studies to get an idea of how many people actually keep the weight off for two or more years. They found that the average weight loss was around two pounds, and that between one third and two thirds of the individuals actually put on more weight than they lost! The authors of the study, led by Traci Mann at the Health and Eating Laboratory at the University of Minnesota, come to the blunt conclusion that dieting simply does not work. Indeed, they suggest that "the most positive conclusion is that dieting slows the slight weight gain that occurs with age among the average non-dieter." Another study of over nine hundred individuals published in the *International Journal of Obesity and Related Metabolic Disorders* found that after fifteen years, only 6 percent had managed to keep off just 5 percent of the initial weight lost, leading the authors to conclude that "long-term weight loss is rare." Is there any reason to think that a cleanse or, for that matter, any trendy new diet, will for some magical reason reverse this trend? No. When you hear about some new approach to dieting, always take this skeptical position. History tells us that the skeptical position will almost always be correct.

You *will* lose weight, temporarily, on a cleanse—as I was clearly doing—but it has absolutely *nothing* to do with the removal of toxins. The weight loss that happens on a cleanse is the direct result of two factors: (1) eating fewer calories and (2) monitoring what you are eating, which leads to eating fewer calories. Okay, it is really the result of one factor: eating fewer calories.

And because many cleanses involve a drastic reduction in calorie intake, the weight often comes off fast. For example, the Master Cleanse—popular with many celebs, including Ashton Kutcher, Ashanti, Pink, and, most famously, Beyoncé in preparation for her role in the movie *Dreamgirls*—is an all-liquid diet based on lemon juice, maple syrup and cayenne pepper. It involves the consumption of six hundred to seven hundred calories a day, which is much less than half the quantity required by an average woman. It is, quite simply, a crash diet.

Is rapid weight loss a bad idea from the perspective of sustained weight maintenance? Here, the data are surprisingly mixed. Intuitively, it seems crazy to put our bodies in starvation mode, slowing the metabolism and, as a result, making it more likely that the weight will come back. Gwyneth herself has made this observation in her well-publicized 2013 critique of the Master Cleanse. (She favours, naturally, Dr. Junger's Clean Cleanse, which allows more calories.) But most of the research suggests that, on its own, rapid weight loss isn't particularly harmful, at least in the context of weight loss and *moderate-term* weight management. (You're wrong again, Gwyneth, even when I want you to be right!) A 2013 review of the relevant literature published in the *New England Journal of Medicine* found that rapid weight loss can be just as effective as slow weight loss. A recent study, published in 2013, supports this view. The study compared the weight-loss success of individuals on 1000- versus 1500-calorie diets and the former fared better, at least after twelve months. (Note: these conclusions do not conflict with the overall weight-loss data. Long-term weight maintenance is *not* the norm. Research has consistently shown that, over time, most dieters struggle to keep weight off.)

Still, the extreme diet approach presents serious problems. First, as the data above highlight, it simply isn't going to work for more than a relatively brief period. If sustained weight loss is your goal, the extreme strategy is destined to fail. I contacted Traci Mann, who is currently a visiting professor at Cambridge University's Institute of Public Health and is working on a book that explores the psychology of dieting, to get her view on the idea of cleansing your way thin. "The fact is, you can lose weight on pretty much any diet in the short term," she says. "But then the weight comes back on. Given that, why put yourself through the discomfort of a cleanse, or any other extreme strategy?" Cleanses are all pain and regain: a lose-lose strategy.

My friend and colleague Dr. Yoni Freedhoff agrees with Mann. He is a weight-loss expert and author of *The Diet Fix*. Freedhoff notes that because cleanses, detoxes and crash diets often focus on a goal, be it a duration (my twenty-one-day cleanse, for instance), a weight or an occasion (such as looking good for your *Vogue* cover photo), failure is almost guaranteed. "Many crash dieters revert to their pre-diet lifestyles," Freedhoff tells me. "Celebrity diets generally fall into what I would describe as traumatic crash diets. Traumatic in that invariably they involve suffering. Crash in that there's a clear end in sight and usually an abrupt one at that." As noted in the *New England Journal of Medicine* article quoted above, "obesity is best concep-tualized as a chronic condition, requiring on-going management to maintain long-term weight loss." Freedhoff could not agree more. "By considering weight as a chronic condition and lifestyle changes as its treatment," he tells me, you can never abandon the treatment or "the weight will return." So, if the maintenance of weight loss is your goal, you'd better like your "treatment." "I've never met anyone who wanted to live on a lemon-pepper cleanse forever," Freedhoff concludes.

If the first problem with cleanse diets is that they don't work, the second problem is that many aren't healthy. They may not, for example, provide adequate nutrients (lemon juice?) and they may erode lean muscle mass. A 2011 study done at the Norwegian Olympic Sport Centre compared the impact of fast and slow weight loss in a group of elite athletes. They found that on all the measured dimensions, including the effect on lean muscle mass, power and strength, the slow weight loss was superior to the fast weight loss. They recommend that athletes aim for about 0.7 percent loss of body weight per week, or about 1.4 pounds if you are a 200-pound man and 1 pound if you are a 150-pound woman.

Ironically, given that improving how you look is so often a key message attached to the marketing of cleanses, some evidence also suggests that cleanse diets may lead to more flab, though the data on this point are inconclusive. At least a few studies have found that repeatedly taking weight off and putting it back on, which is an inevitable consequence of embracing the cleanse approach, is associated with long-term weight gain and the accumulation of abdominal fat. A 2011 study, for example, found that weight cycling, as yo-yo dieting is often called in the academic literature, is associated with a higher than average weight and more abdominal fat as compared to non-yo-yo dieters.

I have absolutely no idea what Anthony Weiner and Brett Favre were thinking. I cannot imagine what would make a man text a picture of his penis to anyone, especially a woman he was trying to win over. Perhaps it had something to do with celebrity ego and the idea that the famous are exempt from normal rules of behavior—a side effect of the assumption of celebrity authority? But the supposed upside is both delusional and implausible. The practice is all risk, no benefit. In fact, it is my belief that all forms of sexting make absolutely no sense.

But I did it anyway. I couldn't stop myself. I just looked so damn good.

It was the last day of my cleanse. I had made it. It was a wretched grind, but things did get a wee bit better after my caffeine withdrawal subsided. Did I feel pure now? I don't think so. Did I feel happy? Only because it was the last day of my cleanse. Did I feel lighter? Yes, I did.

I lost around nine pounds off my already relatively lean body. Nine pounds in three weeks. Not insignificant. *This is the most toned I'll probably ever be*, I mused, as I struck a few muscleman poses for the benefit of no one but my own vain self. And that was when it happened. Without thinking, I grabbed my phone, flexed, snapped a pic in that terrible arm-stretched-out selfie manner and texted it to my wife.

At least, Mr. Weiner, I kept my pants on. It was just a bit of harmless flexting.

WHY SO POPULAR?

Given the sketchy logic and lack of evidence, why are cleanses so popular? I am fascinated by this question, particularly as many reputable and easily accessible sources of health information are unequivocal about the unproven nature of cleanses and detox diets. The Mayo Clinic website, for example, notes that "they're not scientifically proven." And WebMD, one of the single most popular sources for health information, notes that "experts say they are neither necessary nor scientifically proven to work." Yahoo! Health goes even further: "The claims that extreme detoxing will rid your body of toxins, give you more energy and melt away pounds aren't true." But the truth never takes. On the contrary, the popularity of cleanses—and, for that matter, all trendy diets—seems to be growing.

A big part of the story, of course, is that celebrities are vocal supporters of the trend. Celebrities are also under intense pressure to look a certain way. They are both desperate consumers and ardent purveyors of dieting fads. And because they look so darn great, it's easy for the unwary to conclude that cleansing works. But more must be going on. The evidence against the value of trendy diets is just so undeniable and the whole concept so silly, it seems unlikely that celebrity endorsements alone would be enough to keep this pseudoscience thriving.

I asked Walter Willett, professor of epidemiology and nutrition chair for the Department of Nutrition at the Harvard School of Public Health, to speculate about the continued interest in cleansing despite the clear lack of evidence. His guess: "It is possible that taking a break from the steady overeating that is the norm for most Americans could have some benefit and make people feel better."

I think he is onto something. I do think people view cleanses as a break. But I would take it even further than Willett. I am speculating here, but I think one of the reasons cleanses have so much traction is that they are more than just a break: they are viewed, consciously or unconsciously, as a way to pay for our lifestyle sins. Cleanses are like a form of self-flagellation. They are a short-term atonement for bad nutrition choices and consumption excesses. Many celebrities, including Gwyneth, often frame cleanses in these terms—as retribution for holiday indulgences, for example. Gwyneth seems to go on a cleanse every January. ("It is that time of year, folks. I need to lose a few pounds of holiday excess. Anyone else?" she wrote on her Goop website on December 31, 2008.)

Adding to the penance vibe is the reinforcement you get

from friends and even strangers. With few exceptions, they offered me words of encouragement. I got many in the vein of "good for you" and "hang in there." Nobody laughed at me or told me I was nuts. It was generally perceived as a righteous activity, like recycling, driving an electric car or commuting on your bike in the middle of an Edmonton winter. You can also experience a massive sense of accomplishment when you finish. The mountain summited. The marathon completed. So even though the cleanse has no real health benefits, you have a sense that you have done *something*, which likely adds to the placebo effect that leads one to feel pure, happy and clean.

I've experienced this feeling of triumph over starvation before. When I was fourteen my older brother, Case, dared me to stop eating. Actually, it was more of a sibling rivalry–fueled contest than a dare. It was summer vacation. We were bored. And Case was reading *Alive*, the book about the soccer team that crashed in the Andes. The survivors were so desperate for food they ate their dead teammates; hence my brother's no-food fixation. Case figured we should give it a try—going without food, that is, not eating human flesh. The rules for our little game were simple: whoever went the longest without food won the contest.

I wish I could report that I outlasted my big bro, but alas, it was a tie. After two full days and much moaning and quarreling, we came to a mutual agreement to stop. (It is hard to imagine a parent of the current hyper-vigilant variety allowing this to continue beyond morning snack time. It was a different time, as they say.) I vividly remember three things about this tournament. First, I really thought two days without calories was a significant achievement. Second, the first thing I ate when we threw in the towel was an entire row of Chips Ahoy cookies, which I am fairly certain would not be a Gwyneth-approved post-cleanse strategy. And third, and this is the reason I relate this story, I got a buzz out of the experience.

The popularity of cleansing may be tied to this kind of psychological pick-me-up. It has been noted in some clinical studies that individuals in the first stages of starvation often experience a heightened sense of well-being or bliss. (Note: during my Gwyneth-inspired cleanse I never felt anything close to euphoric or blissful, or even well.) For those who experience it, the sensation may be the result of the release of endorphins associated with extreme calorie restriction. Starvation will do that.

Of course, the other reason cleanses are so popular is that they lead to short-term weight loss. I lost weight. Again, starvation will do that.

THE NO-GIMMICK CLEANSE

Perhaps I should simply stop fighting it: people want a cleanse. If you can't beat them, join them, as they say. So, here is the Caulfield Cleanse. It is simple. It is cheap. In fact, it might save you money. You don't need to buy any useless supplements, vitamins or special juices. You don't need to consume fancy powder drinks or avoid gluten, coffee or even (moderate) amounts of alcohol. And I guarantee it will work.

Step 1: Cleanse your system of all the pseudoscience babble that flows from many celebrities, celebrity physicians and the diet industry.

Step 2: Supplement with a daily dose of healthy skepticism.

Step 3: Detoxify your system with evidence produced by the scientific community and disseminated by independent entities (a favorite source: The Cochrane Collaboration).

Step 4: Watch your calorie intake (diet diaries are a terrific and evidence-based strategy) and eat lots of fruits and vegetables (aim for about 50 percent of what goes in your mouth).

I am only half joking. Virtually every science-informed expert I contacted said the same thing. People should forget about cleanses and trendy diets and concentrate on consuming an appropriate number of calories (for most, this is between 1800 and 2200 per day) and eating in a nutritious manner, which means fruits, vegetables, whole grains, nuts, legumes, lean protein (including fish) and a bit of dairy. In fact, the preceding sentence captures almost all you need to know about a healthy diet. You can ignore everything else.

While a healthy diet consists of more than just fruits and vegetables, this is a logical place to start. If we could just increase the percentage of people who eat an adequate amount of fruits and vegetables, we could have a real, long-term impact on the health of the population. Few of us eat enough of these foods. Research from the United States says that, in 2009, fewer than 14 percent of people ate the recommended amount. And a 2013 study from Sweden involving more than seventy thousand participants found that eating fruits and vegetables was associated with a longer and healthier life. Another massive study, also from 2013, followed almost half a million people and found a similar reduction of mortality, particularly in the context of cardiovascular disease. Other recent research has found that fruits and vegetables may protect against mental health issues and assist with sustained weight maintenance. Also, making this conscious effort to consume more fruits and veggies may allow people to feel like they are committing to a fresh start or "resetting" their system, two concepts that seem central to the popularity of the cleansing strategy.

So, keep it simple. Ignore the hype. Remember, history tells us all dieting trends are likely to be wrong. They never work. Below are just a few examples of topics and trends that are distorted by celebrity culture's spin.

Coffee: "Today I quit my beloved coffee & make the switch to vitamin B complex," Katy Perry told the world via Twitter. Why would anyone quit coffee for health reasons? Coffee is *good* for you. No evidence suggests that coffee exhausts your adrenals or is taxing your detox organs (sigh), as the cleansing gurus of the world would have us believe. And lots of evidence indicates that it protects against a variety of ailments, including Parkinson's, type 2 diabetes and liver cancer. It also improves brain function and athletic performance. Drink up, Ms. Perry. Coffee is making you healthier. (Full disclosure, my deep love of coffee may impact my interpretation of the data, despite my halfhearted effort to remain semi-objective on this matter.)

Vitamins and supplements: What about Ms. Perry's much-publicized decision to start consuming a boatload of vitamins? In May 2013, for example, she tweeted a picture of herself to her then forty-six million followers holding up three massive bags of pills, which, apparently, she gulps down upon rising, with breakfast and at dinner. "I'm all about that supplement & vitamin LYFE!" she said.

In fact, most studies suggest that taking vitamins and supplements—which I was required to do as part of my cleanse—is usually completely unnecessary and might even be harmful. A study of almost forty thousand women, for instance, found no benefit to taking a range of supplements and concluded that there was "little justification for the general and widespread use of dietary supplements." Research has also found that vitamin C does not prevent cancer or, for that matter, colds; supplementation with some vitamins (e.g., A and E) may increase the risk of certain cancers; taking supplements with omega-3 may increase the risk of prostate cancer; and, to quote a document from the Harvard School of Public Health, further supplementation with high doses of the vitamin Bs "has not been found to be beneficial and might actually cause harm."

Other studies have discovered that many supplements are often not what they say they are. Indeed, chances are Ms. Perry has no idea what she is gobbling in her attempt to live a healthier LYFE. A 2013 study from the University of Guelph, for example, did a blind study of commercially available supplements and found that "most of the herbal products were of poor quality, including considerable product substitution, contamination and use of fillers." Remarkably, they found some product substitution—the use of another, unlabeled herb in place of the main ingredient—in products of 83 percent of the companies tested. In other words, only 17 percent of the companies were providing products that matched what the label said. This is, of course, both dangerous and unethical. It should not be forgotten that the massive supplement and vitamin industry, worth, by some estimates, approximately $60 billion worldwide, is about profits and moving product. Because of the bucks to be made, many pharmaceutical companies have recently acquired companies that produce supplements. Since it is not a tightly regulated industry, this situation should surprise no one.

You should strive to get all your vitamins from the food you eat, not from pills. Even in the context of vitamin D, a supplement that has received a lot of attention in the popular press, the evidence is more equivocal than often portrayed. A 2010 report from the US Institute of Medicine (IOM) of the National Academies of Science found that while vitamin D plays a key role in bone health, most of us get enough via food and sun. It reported that current evidence "does not support other benefits of vitamin D" intake and that the higher levels associated with supplement intake may be harmful. So more is not better. A more recent analysis, published in 2013 by the US Preventive Services Task Force, found that even in the context of bone health, insufficient evidence exists about the benefits of vitamin D supplements to recommend their use for most populations. A subsequent study, published in late 2013 in the journal *The Lancet*, has taken it even further, finding that vitamin D is not necessary for bone health in otherwise healthy individuals. And yet another study, this one from 2014 and published in *The Lancet Diabetes & Endocrinology*, concluded that vitamin D had little effect on a range of health problems, including cardiovascular disease, mood disorders and weight gain. The lead author of the study was quoted in *The New York Times*, thus: "Unfortunately, there is probably no benefit to expect from vitamin D supplementation in normally healthy people."

I am not saying that there is never a reason to take a supplement. Pregnant women, for example, have particular needs and some individuals may have clear, clinically determined deficiencies. And data on some supplements, such as vitamin D, are still being compiled. But to date, absolutely no evidence indicates that living a "supplement & vitamin LYFE" is a good idea. Most of the relevant science suggests the opposite.

Colon cleanses: The idea that a colon cleanse removes toxins and promotes health is so ridiculous that it is a pretty good test for quacks. If a book, health care practitioner, TV doctor, magazine columnist and/or blogger recommends a colon cleanse, also known as a colonic or colonic hydrotherapy, you can flush all their advice down the toilet.

On this subject, I don't need to mince words. Colon cleanses don't work and are potentially harmful. Even though celebs including Madonna, Leonardo DiCaprio and Britney Spears may have embraced the fecal flush, the whole concept is nonsense. As noted in a 2011 review of the relevant scientific literature, there are "no scientifically robust studies in support of this practice." Other reviews have come to a similar conclusion. Not only does it do no good, the practice is also likely to be harmful. It can result in nausea, vomiting, infection and, in rare circumstances, perforation of the bowel. It can also adversely impact your electrolytes and your gut's natural bacteria. All of these potential risks are, of course, increased the more frequently you do colon cleanses.

Incidentally, in his book *Clean*, Dr. Junger recommends colonic hydrotherapy—which is, as he explains, "the injection of pure water delivered at low pressure into the colon and then drawn out." He further advises thus: "You can have as many [colonic] treatments during Clean as you like, depending on your budget and schedule. (I've even had patients who got them daily during their detox.)" I'll leave it to you to determine the degree to which the recommendation of daily colon cleanses impacts his credibility.

While I followed all the rules associated with my Clean Cleanse, I could not bring myself to implement this part of the program. Unnecessary. Unsafe. Unscientific. And kind of disgusting.

Juicing: Forbes recently called juicing a "Celebrity Trend Gone Wild." Which, given the huge increase in the sale of both premade juices and home juicing machines, is a more than fair assessment. If you Google Image "celebrity juicing," you get pictures of Hilary Duff, Jennifer Garner, Nicole Richie, Orlando Bloom, Blake Lively, Olivia Wilde and, of course, Gwyneth holding some kind of (usually green) juice concoction.

The premise behind juicing is that by removing the harder-to-digest fiber (many of the trending juices are "pressed") the vitamins will be concentrated and easier to digest. The problem is that, once again, no evidence supports the concept that juicing is a better way to get our fruits and vegetables, lose weight, remove toxins or ingest calories. I also could not find a cogent explanation as to why we need to absorb our vitamins quickly—presuming, of course, that juicing allows this to happen—or give our digestive tract a break from fiber. Indeed, studies have found that drinking your calories is far from ideal because liquids don't make humans feel as full as solid foods. Think about how you feel after eating an actual apple, banana and half a cup of blueberries, and compare that to how you feel after drinking juice with the same ingredients. Not the same. A study from 2013 concluded that people find solid meals more satisfying than liquids—even meal-replacement shakes. (No surprise here, given my experience with the less-than-gratifying Clean Cleanse shakes.) Other studies have shown that the consumption of liquid instead of solid calories is associated with increased calorie intake and higher body mass index (BMI).

A 2013 investigation by the Harvard School of Public Health confirmed the tremendous benefits of eating an adequate amount of fruits and vegetables, but, once again, found juice to be problematic. The research looked at data from almost 190,000 participants and found that individuals who ate whole fruits—especially blueberries, grapes and apples—reduced their risk for type 2 diabetes by 23 percent. But individuals who drank one or two servings of fruit juice actually *increased* their risk. So, put down that expensive, trendy, kale-infused liquid and pick up a real apple.

Okay, to be fair, unlike colonics, there is nothing inherently dangerous about juicing or the closely related smoothie. (Smoothies probably are slightly better for you, because they are usually made by blending the entire fruit and, as a result, include more fiber—but the juicing/smoothie jargon is a bit slippery.) And, I suppose, juicing can be a way to get a more varied intake of fruits and vegetables. But neither is there anything magically healthy about juicing or juice products. Unless some medical reason prevents you from masticating—perhaps a paparazzo's camera broke your jaw?—juicing shouldn't be viewed as a nutrition strategy. This fad is based on such a thin rationale that it may fade soon. Indeed, the whole juicing scene is getting pretty wacky. "All our juices are handcrafted—it's more of an art," one New York juicing company owner was quoted as saying in the New York *Daily News*. When people start talking about "handcrafted" juice, we are nearing the point where Fonzie is warming up the speedboat in preparation for his jump over a cold-pressed, organic juice–filled shark tank.

Organic: This one is tough. I need to tread carefully or the hate mail will flow. It is a complex topic and many feel passionate about eating organic. As usual, of course, celebs lead the way. "I find the most satisfying food is food that's full of life, so it's raw and clean and organic," says model Miranda Kerr. And, naturally, Gwyneth and Dr. Junger are big on organic. The word "organic" appears often on the pages of the Clean Cleanse manual (actual count: twelve mentions in a forty-eight-page document).

But despite the deep attachment that many individuals and organizations have to organic food, the evidence about its benefits is far from conclusive. The best available research suggests that organic food—which, by the way, can be tough to define—is not nutritionally superior to conventionally grown products. Given that studies tell us that personal health is a key reason that people buy organic, and given the enthusiasm with which they endorse the practice, it is important to note that this is the conclusion formed by numerous respected organizations and researchers. For example, in 2009 the UK Food Standards Agency did a meta-analysis of the scientific evidence and found "no evidence of a health benefit from consuming organic compared to conventionally produced foodstuffs." A more recent study, published in 2012 by a team from Stanford University, agreed, noting that no strong evidence indicates that "organic foods are significantly more nutritious than conventional foods."

Some studies have found that some organic foods have slightly more micronutrients and less pesticide residue, but, despite these findings, no good studies "have directly demonstrated health benefits or disease protection as a result of consuming an organic diet," to quote a review published in the journal *Pediatrics* in 2012. In other words, even if small differences do exist, no evidence suggests these differences are clinically relevant. Indeed, most of the available data suggest they are not—but, to be fair, more research on this point would be helpful. (The micronutrient concern seems a bit ridiculous. The differences, if any exist, are so small that a tiny additional bite of a conventionally grown item would more than compensate.) It should also be recognized that organic farming also uses pesticides, though only "natural" ones. But this doesn't mean they are necessarily healthier or better for the environment. To quote Steven Novella from a piece written for *Evidence-Based Medicine*, "There is little to no evidence that these organic pesticides are less harmful for consumers or the environment. It is just assumed that they are based upon the naturalistic fallacy." While not all will agree with this opinion (I do!), it is important to recognize the scientific uncertainty about the supposed benefits of organic food. Here is just one example that highlights the uncertainty: a University of Guelph study from 2010 found that "organic approved insecticides had a similar or even greater negative impact on several natural enemy species in lab studies, were more detrimental to biological control organisms in field experiments, and had higher [environmental impact] at field use rates."

A recent analysis by the Canadian government found that almost 50 percent of organic food has residue from synthetic pesticides. One of the government officials quoted in the story, which was reported in January 2014, suggests that this level of contamination likely indicates deliberate use of synthetic pesticides by some organic farmers.

Despite what the science tells us, people will, no doubt, continue to purchase organic products. Buying organic food is, like many purchasing choices, as much a way of expressing a worldview—or even a form of self-expression—as it is a diet choice. People buy organic for many reasons, including taste, concern about the environment and a desire to help the local economy. For some, it is also associated with a desire to represent a particular alternative, anti-corporate lifestyle. Two ironic twists emerge from this personal-branding side of organic food. First, organic food is now a huge, multibillion-dollar industry that preys on and profits from the consumer's desire to project a particular healthy and environmentally friendly ethos. Big Food companies such as Kellogg and PepsiCo now own many organic food brands. As noted in a 2012 *New York Times* article that outlined the corporatization of organic food (or, as the author calls it, Big Organic), "Pure, locally produced ingredients from small family farms? Not so much anymore." Second, an interesting and, to be honest, kind of funny study explored the degree to which purchasing organic food impacted moral attitudes and altruistic behavior. Given the degree to which organic food is marketed with moral overtones—organic brands have names such as Honest Team, Purity Life, Seeds of Change, Living Tree Community—the author was curious about whether organic food had an impact on how people behaved. The study came to the paradoxical conclusion that being exposed to organic food does not make individuals into caring, open-minded hippies. It makes people more self-righteous, judgmental and *less* altruistic. This admittedly small study led an editor at *The Atlantic* magazine to ask, "Does Organic Food Make You a Judgmental Jerk?" For me, it highlights the complex relationship between food and our beliefs. What we eat both reflects and, perhaps, shapes how we see the world.

If you enjoy the taste of organic food (although numerous studies have found little evidence to support the "tastes better" claim, including a 2012 study that found blinded consumers actually preferred the taste of *conventionally* grown tomatoes!) or like the idea of buying your food at a farmers' market, then, by all means, carry on. (Hey! I do it too!) But do not believe any of the rhetoric that suggests you'll reap additional health benefits. Don't believe the claims that conventional foods contain fatigue-generating toxins or that they will exhaust your adrenals. Absolutely no good evidence exists to show that this is true.

Gluten: Near the beginning of the movie *This Is the End*, Seth Rogen, playing himself, tells his buddy Jay Baruchel that "he is on a cleanse" and that we should all stop eating gluten. "Whenever you feel shitty, that's because of gluten," Rogen explains. "Gluten is a vague term. It's something that's used to categorize things that are bad. Ya know? Calories, that's a gluten. Fat, that's a gluten." It is a hilarious scene. And it is spot on. The bit captures the current insanity surrounding gluten and, more broadly, wheat, which have become the new food devils. Every conceivable human health problem has been attributed to the consumption of gluten and/or wheat, including fatigue, obesity, diabetes, migraines, Alzheimer's and even autism. (This last one has been pushed by, no surprise here, Jenny McCarthy.)

The demonization of gluten, which is a protein found in wheat and other grains, can be traced to bestselling books such as *Wheat Belly* and, naturally, advocacy by hordes of gluten-free celebrities, including Gwyneth and Steve Nash. Gluten-free has become a massive industry. Some estimates put the size of the gluten-free food market at around $6 billion, as approximately 20 percent of the population now buys gluten-free products. The primary reasons for the popularity of this diet approach are, first, the belief that it is healthier and, second, that it will lead to weight loss. Indeed, a survey of more than two hundred dietitians pegged gluten-free as 2013's most popular diet and weight-loss approach.

But what does the relevant science say?

Unfortunately, the evidence does not provide straightforward answers. Let's start with the facts that seem pretty certain. Despite claims to the contrary, no credible study has shown that gluten/wheat is the cause of the current obesity epidemic. Also, no credible evidence suggests that going gluten- and wheat-free is a wise lifestyle choice—unless, of course, you have a clinically identified reason for doing so (for example, if you are one of the approximately 1 percent who have celiac disease). Nor is it a proven weight-loss strategy. In fact, some studies have found that going gluten-free can lead to weight gain. A 2006 study, for example, followed 371 gluten-free dieters—these were individuals with celiac disease—and found that 82 percent gained weight after two years. Not so surprising, perhaps, given that we have no reason to assume gluten-free food has fewer calories.

One review article nicely summarized the research on this point: "It is important to note that gluten-free does not necessarily mean low-energy, and some gluten-free products actually have a greater energy value than corresponding gluten-containing foods."

Many anecdotal reports of gluten-free weight-loss success have appeared in the media, often connected to some super-slim celeb. For example, a 2013 article in the *Daily Mail* headlined "Gluten-free devotee Miley Cyrus shows off her flat stomach" tells us that the "bread, pasta and pizza-free way of life seems to be paying off for Miley Cyrus."

Ignore this kind of hype. Anecdotes and personal testimonials—no matter how compelling and belly-button revealing—are not good science. The evidence tells us that whole grains are actually good for us. They are, among other things, full of fiber and vitamins. Studies have consistently found that the healthiest diets, such as the Mediterranean diet, contain whole grains.

It seems likely that much of the gluten-free craze is the result of celebrity culture and opportunistic marketing. Gluten-free products are generally expensive and, one can assume, highly profitable. A recent editorial in the *British Medical Journal* goes so far as to suggest that the entire area is "being driven by profit and market forces, not medical forces." As a 2011 consumer information document published by the US Food and Drug Administration put it, "For people not sensitive to gluten, there is no health benefit to a gluten-free diet."

Okay, so going gluten-free isn't a smart weight-loss or nutrition strategy, but what about the ever-increasing number of people who report sensitivity to gluten? I want to emphasize, again, that I am not referring to individuals who have celiac disease, which is a condition that can be diagnosed through laboratory tests. For people with this relatively rare condition, avoiding gluten is necessary. Here, I am referring to individuals who do not have celiac disease but still feel that gluten is causing symptoms such as stomach pain, diarrhea, bloating and fatigue. This is where things get a bit confusing.

On one side of the argument is the dubious nature of the evidence. For example, no definitive biomarkers (e.g., blood tests, tissue samples, etc.) are associated with gluten sensitivity and the best studies have failed to clearly identify the condition. This has led many researchers to question the very existence of non-celiac gluten sensitivity. A recent study from Australia, for example, used a sophisticated double-blind approach (i.e., neither the researchers nor the research participants knew whether the food was truly gluten-free) and found no evidence of gluten sensitivity. An editorial accompanying the study, which was published in the journal *Gastroenterology*, suggests the "study calls into question the very existence of NCGS [non-celiac gluten sensitivity] as a discrete entity."

I contacted two of the study's authors, Jessica Biesiekierski and Peter Gibson, from the Department of Gastroenterology at Monash University in Australia. Both have been researching this issue for years. The results, as Peter Gibson told me, were pretty definitive. "Our recent study using the 'gold standard' of repeated double-blinded placebo-controlled re-challenge showed in a population of patients who believed they were gluten sensitive that none really were." To repeat, *none* of them were. Naturally, even a definitive finding like this does little to convert believers. You can sense Gibson's frustration. "The take [on this study] by some was that we picked the wrong patients and that we got it wrong in some way. In other words, pseudo-science is more reliable than real science."

Biesiekierski agrees with Gibson but concedes that the growth in self-reported sensitivity hints that something may be going on. "I think there is *some* evidence that NCGS *may* exist, but probably only in a *very small number* of people. However, I am still skeptical and ultimately the existence of NCGS will remain unsubstantiated until there is more definitive, reproducible research."

Some medical researchers have speculated that people feel better when they go gluten-free simply because they start eating better (e.g., more fruits and vegetables) and less. On the other side of the argument are the studies that have tried to map the incidence of gluten sensitivity. Dr. Alessio Fasano from the Center for Celiac Research at Massachusetts General, for example, using both self-report and clinical investigations, has suggested that as much as 6 percent of the population could have some degree of sensitivity. A more recent study from Columbia University put that incidence at a much lower 0.55 percent. But neither conclusion appears to be definitive, and the academic debate about the nature and incidence of gluten sensitivity seems likely to rage for years to come. The bottom line: the science on non-celiac gluten sensitivity is still emerging. As another review of the relevant research, published in September 2013, put it: "Non-celiac gluten sensitivity is an entity awaiting validation, better diagnostic criteria, and, if it does exist, pathogenic mechanisms."

So Seth Rogen was right: gluten is a pretty vague term. Still, the bulk of the science tells us that most of us do not need to shy away from gluten or wheat. Whatever Gwyneth and Miley may tell you, the science doesn't agree.

THREE WEEKS AFTER MY CLEANSE

All of the weight is back on my old, flabby frame. Infuriating. No more flexting. Phone stays in pocket.

CHAPTER 2

BEAUTY TIPS FROM BEAUTIFUL PEOPLE

"Your facial routine is pretty time consuming," my wife, Joanne, says to me as I carefully apply my moisturizing sunscreen, the last phase of my morning skin-care and anti-aging program. It is early, she needs to get to work and she obviously doesn't appreciate my meticulous rinsing procedure. Chop, chop! Let's get a move on!

Until recently, my approach to skin care had been exceedingly time-efficient. It included precisely nothing. Zip. I washed my face with plain, cheap, bulk-purchased soap, which I used only when there was something on my face that needed washing. I didn't even use shaving cream. I just dragged a crappy disposable razor over some of that plain soap. I rarely wore a hat when outside (bad) and almost never put on sunscreen (very bad). But I am a changed man. Twice daily my old skin is now pampered like the Stanley Cup—game seven, third period.

Not long ago I flew to Calgary to meet with an old friend and respected dermatologist, Kirk Barber, now professor in the Faculty of Medicine at the University of Calgary. I met Kirk when I was an undergrad, nearly thirty years ago, and consequently he has seen me at my sartorial worst. I believe the day of our first encounter I sported a fauxhawk, a dangly lightning-bolt earring and a too-tight biker jacket. All things considered, I figured I couldn't do anything to further humiliate myself in his eyes. This makes him the perfect confidant for my latest vanity project. More importantly, he is well positioned to help me sift through all the myths and truths about skin-care and anti-aging practices.

I told Kirk that I wanted to adopt a typical skin-care routine, something that an aging celebrity might use on a daily basis. My goal was both to experience a comprehensive skin-care regime (something I hadn't attempted since I stressed about acne in high school) and to determine whether, in fact, a high-tech routine can make a difference. Are beauty products worth it? Since I was interested in experiencing what people actually do to protect and enhance their skin—and not, necessarily, what the evidence says we *should* be doing—Kirk introduced me to Marie, who ran a "skin science" clinic next to his office. This was not a medical office, but a clinic that provides cosmetic services and products aimed at helping people enhance the look and condition of their skin. "I am, really, a skin coach," Marie told me as she showed me around the office. She has a graduate degree in microbiology, is infectiously good-natured and has absolutely flawless skin.

Marie invited me into her all-white office. White table, white walls, white chairs and white machinery. I told her about my project and hinted that I was pretty skeptical about the whole skin-care industry. She ignored the implied criticism and launched into a heartfelt lecture on the benefits of various products and skin-care routines. She also had a great deal to say about the condition of my skin. Not good. Using a machine that would be at home on the bridge of the starship

Enterprise—the new, J.J. Abrams–directed Enterprise, not the old TV, cardboardy-looking ship—she took a picture of my face that, she explained, would provide a host of information about the treatment she would recommend.

The machine produces a series of colorful, and less-than-flattering, images of my face, each highlighting a particular skin property, such as wrinkles, redness, sun damage and low pore quality. Now, this machine looked impressive, but despite a good bit of digging I could not find an independent analysis of its clinical value. The website for the company that manufactures the machine states, among other things, that the company has "deployed their complexion analysis software as a sales tool to promote" brands of cosmetic products; that it has been shown to "impressively increase business in all of your skin care services"; and that it "was never intended for clinical trials." Reading between the lines (or, actually, simply reading the lines), it seems the company views this machine as a way to move product. So there are reasons to be skeptical about the meaning and relevance of the results. Still, the premise of the device—taking pictures of my face to assess its condition—is not farfetched. I go with the flow.

The good news: my wrinkle situation is great. For my age and ethnicity, I have fewer wrinkles than about 95 percent of the population. It must be all that plain, bulk-purchased soap. The bad news: my pore situation is catastrophic. The picture reveals that I have over one thousand clogged pores on my face. "You have the worst pores I have seen in over eight years," Marie tells me with a shake of her head. I stifle the sudden impulse to dash out of the room to scrub my filthy face with an industrial-strength solvent.

To be honest, I have never noticed and no one has ever commented on my poor-pore predicament. My wife has never mentioned it. Nor have my singularly candid children and brothers ever mocked me about it. Nevertheless, according to the picture produced by Marie's Star Trek machine, this was a serious cosmetic problem that needed fixing. I left Marie's office with a bag full of high-end beauty products, including a cleansing/exfoliation gel that was designed to decongest aging skin, another cleansing lotion to control bacteria, a nighttime moisturizer that claims to be specifically designed for bad pores and a morning moisturizer that doubles as a sunblock. The plan was to use these products morning and night for three months.

BIG BEAUTY AND THE EVIDENCE CHALLENGE

The beauty industry is, of course, massive. It involves everything from teeth-whitening toothpaste to ridiculously expensive shampoo that will transform your hair (to quote an advertisement for a product that contains white truffles and caviar and costs more than $60 for an 8.5 oz bottle) "from ordinary to extraordinary." It involves celebrity-endorsed cosmetics, perfumes and a host of fashion products. And it involves numerous fitness and slimming gimmicks. I will make no attempt to undertake a comprehensive analysis of every allegedly beautifying product that is touched by a celebrity. Their number is infinite. It's enough to know that the beauty industry is a huge cultural force in a tight, symbiotic relationship with celebrities and the celebrity-oriented media. The size and influence of this industry creates challenges for anyone seeking to get to the truth about the products it makes and promotes.

In my research I worked hard to find experts who could provide a reasonably independent view about the alleged benefits of the myriad beauty and anti-aging products and services. This proved to be much more difficult than I anticipated. Many of the experts I contacted were not independent scientists but dermatologists who also had a clinical practice and, as such, benefit (some, greatly) from a thriving industry. I am *not* saying that physicians knowingly twist information about the efficacy of beauty treatments, but ample evidence suggests that this kind of conflict of interest can have an impact on how research is presented and interpreted.

In addition, very little independent literature exists on the subject. For many beauty products, either no data or only small studies that are produced by the proponents of the product exists. To some degree, this is understandable. Government research entities, such as the US National Institutes of Health or the Canadian Institutes of Health Research, have little interest in funding big double-blind placebo-controlled trials on the efficacy, for instance, of bird-poop facial cream. So not a lot of good science is available to draw on. To make matters worse, the popular press is rarely critical of new beauty products. While I found many excellent and balanced media stories on beauty treatments (usually panning them), the vast majority of articles simply trumpet their alleged value, using vague descriptors such as "revitalize" and "radiate." Real evidence or expertise rarely appears, beyond personal testimonies (which I don't need to remind you are not evidence). The "experts" who are quoted in these articles are often part of the beauty industry or individuals with no research background. To cite just one example, a frequently quoted "expert" who is a beauty columnist for a well-known women's health magazine and an advocate for all things pseudoscientific, describes herself as an eco-advisor, television personality and restaurateur—interesting résumé, for sure, but hardly a background that lends itself to a critical analysis of beauty products. And remember, publishers don't generally sell magazines by reminding readers that nothing works. And they're unlikely to make a practice of denigrating the industry that purchases so much of their advertising space. So they have a built-in tendency to recommend beauty products by either explicitly or implicitly suggesting that they work.

Consequently, getting straight answers about anti-aging and beauty products is nearly impossible. There exists a confluence of fact-twisting forces: lots of money to be made by manufacturers and providers, huge advertising campaigns that deploy vast quantities of pseudoscientific gobbledygook, a lack of independent research and information, and consumers who desperately want the products to do for them what is claimed. The cumulative impact of all these forces results in a massive bias toward representing a product or procedure as effective. Let's call this the "beauty industry efficacy bias" or the BIEB for short. Sadly, very few social forces push back on the other side of the BIEB equation, so the BIEB reigns supreme. (Note: the link between the BIEB acronym and Justin Bieber's nickname was not intentional—honest!—but it does work well. This struggling singer occupies a hefty hunk of the celebrity culture space and has endorsed a variety of beauty products.)

Given the existence of the BIEB, we should always bring a furiously critical eye to the assessment of any claim made by Big Beauty. Phrases such as "clinically proven" or "dermatologist approved" have little meaning because they could refer to almost anything. For example, what kind of study led to the representation that a given product was clinically proven? Did the manufacturers simply ask a couple of patients? Do not be fooled by this kind of language, particularly when the presence of the BIEB makes critical analysis of the claims unlikely.

In addition to the BIEB dilemma, history tells us that a skeptical position is almost always correct. As with trendy diets, after the passage of a bit of time it almost invariably becomes clear that the alleged benefits associated with some new, exciting anti-aging beauty product can't live up to the hype.

CELEBRITY SKIN, CELEBRITY SOLUTIONS

"I'll have the omelet," I tell the waiter. "Excellent choice," he replies.

I'm sitting on the porch of a Beverly Hills restaurant called The Ivy with the singular purpose of looking for celebrity skin. Facial skin, that is. I am in the Hollywood area, I'm researching celebrity dermatological routines and I figure I might as well get a look at the real deal. I want to compare my normal-person epidermis to the unique and otherworldly qualities of a face that has been properly pampered. Do celebrities really radiate? Do they glow? I figure that The Ivy is my best bet because it is a well-known hangout for celebs. As one Los Angeles travel website notes, "The attention-hungry frequently sit on the front patio, where only a white picket fence separates them from prying lenses." That is exactly where I am sitting and, as luck would have it, the prying lenses are about eight feet away.

Sitting at a table in front of me is a group of beautiful

young women. They are attracting a gaggle of photographers, so, I am guessing, one or more of them must be reasonably famous. While I like to believe that I am in touch with popular culture, I have absolutely no idea who they are. One looks vaguely familiar—perhaps she's a model?—but I can't place her. I desperately want to snap a picture for future research, but the waiter has told me to put away both my phone and computer. (For some reason, the producer-sounding guy sitting nearby is allowed to keep his electronics in plain view. *Do I have a stalker vibe?*) I manage to sneak a picture of my outrageously delicious omelet—which was only slightly less expensive than a slab of plutonium—but no picture of customers opposite. These women, who look young enough to be in high school, do indeed have categorically impeccable skin. Flawless. I might even detect a slight glow.

Just as I get perilously close to a staring intensity that I fear will attract we-must-ask-you-to-leave attention, one of the women starts primping. She is fussing with her hair, applying stuff to her lips, etc. She then pops up from her chair and starts posing for the paparazzi. Hand on hip. Hair fling. Over the shoulder. Big smile. Sexy smile. Pouty face. The cameras snap obediently in response. This goes on for about a minute, and then a waiter dolefully shoos the photographers away. The young woman plops back into her seat and continues chatting with her friends as if nothing has happened. It almost seemed staged. Perhaps it was.

I realize this is an utterly silly experiment. Of course twenty-something model-type women, and probably most of humanity, have skin superior to my blotchy, clogged Celtic hide. I didn't really expect to find any dermatologically challenged celebrities. But the incident perfectly frames the role of celebrity culture in the realm of beauty. The beauty standard set by celebrity culture and the beauty industry is often calibrated by just the kind of photographer–celebrity interaction I witnessed while inhaling an overpriced brunch. Young women posing for pictures.

In many ways, celebrity culture sits at the center of the massive skin-care and anti-aging industry. Some estimates put the global skin-care market at approximately $80 billion, and it has been suggested that the entire anti-aging industry will be worth almost $300 billion by 2015. Celebrity culture helps to set the benchmark for how our skin is supposed to look. (In a word: young—as nicely illustrated by my neighbors at The Ivy.) Celebrities are increasingly used to market skin-care products. And through their well-publicized beauty rituals they help to perpetuate an assortment of anti-aging and skin-care beliefs— the vast majority of which are unscientific and completely unproven.

Celebrities are at once the victims and generators of beauty myths. They primp for paparazzi, thus helping to create the standard by which we are all measured. But, having set the standard, they must also strive to maintain it. People in the entertainment industry, especially women, are under unbelievable pressure to appear young. I heard this message over and over from directors and actors and from the dermatologists who work with them. This being the case, we should, I suppose, cut celebrities a bungee-cord length of slack when it comes to their choice of beauty regimens. Desperation can obscure rational reflection and prompt experimentation with anything that might help to maintain a "youthful" glow.

But the beauty-regimen quackery is hard to take when the pseudoscientific mumbo jumbo is peddled to the masses via interviews, endorsements and celebrity gossip. The popular press usually presents this stuff without a scintilla of critical analysis. On the contrary. At times a mocking tone is discernible—it is tough to report on David and Victoria Beckham's use of bird-poo facials without at least a hint of tongue-in-cheekness—but more often than not, the beauty products are presented as new, exciting and effective. This is the BIEB at work.

A cursory scan of popular newspapers and magazines turns up an overwhelming number of questionable celebrity beauty tips. Virtually every magazine with a focus on fashion, celebrities, health or fitness offers regular advice on skin care and anti-aging. Most newspapers have a weekly style or beauty section. At any given moment, probably hundreds of beauty-related recommendations are available on the average mid-size magazine stand. And all of these stories are almost completely devoid of any reference to credible evidence. Beauty advice is a science-free zone. Anything goes.

It is no surprise, then, that celebrity anti-aging activities, whether mildly nutty or utterly senseless, usually evade informed scrutiny. For example, it was reported in many newspapers and magazines—most without a single reference to science—that Kate Middleton used a bee-venom facial as a needle-free shortcut to youthful, line-free skin. (Isn't the princess *already*, chronologically speaking, pretty darn "youthful"?) I read numerous stories about celebrities using placental face masks, which were described as coming from some ultra-pure sheep in the mountains of New Zealand. Not one of these stories questioned the effectiveness of the sheep afterbirth as an anti-aging ointment, and several said it worked. A similarly uncritical attitude characterized stories about Demi Moore's famous leech therapy (which, as one source states, "cleanses the blood, improves circulation and boosts tissue healing") and the use of snails on the face, favored by celebs such as Katie Holmes, a method that, as reported by *Glamour*, leaves a trail of "mucus that's packed with proteins, antioxidants, and hyaluronic acid, which leave the skin looking glowy and refreshed." Apparently, the face-crawling gastropods are fed only organic vegetables (not making that up).

I found the snail story particularly ridiculous. It got full-page treatment in my local newspaper, which featured a large picture of a young, wrinkle-free model with snails on her face. The story contained a bunch of scientific-sounding jargon—pushing the idea that snail slime has the same cocktail of "beauty-boosting" (could there be a more ambiguous term?) ingredients mentioned in the article about Katie Holmes. The only "experts" quoted were a beauty salon employee ("Slime from snails helps remove old cells, heal the skin ... and moisturize it.") and the sales manager for the salon peddling the service. This wasn't a news story: it was an advertisement. While I am sure snail slime can help make the skin look "glowy" (gooey might be a more apt term), I could find no evidence to support any of the anti-aging and beauty-boosting claims. In case you are interested, the sixty-minute snail treatment costs $240 and is called (again, I am not making this up) the Celebrity Escargot Course.

I realize that most of us don't take these kinds of stories too seriously. They are fun and entertaining diversions. Only a small segment of the public is willing to pay the ridiculous prices demanded by their purveyors for purifying snails, placenta material, insect poison and nightingale excrement. But these stories help to frame how we think about beauty, and they foster the illusion that celebrity status provides access to magically effective anti-aging treatments. They make it seem as if something *can* be done.

But in addition to these extreme beauty treatments, many other stories about anti-aging routines seem both less farfetched and more accessible. These are the treatments that have gone mainstream, thanks in part to celebrity endorsements. Among the most widely known are regimens involving hydration, acupuncture, coffee and a variety of spa treatments. I'll examine all four, but first, a word about words.

Several expressions appear over and over again where beauty products are promoted. These words and phrases sound great, but they're vague, unquantifiable and, if we are honest with ourselves, pretty meaningless. I suspect that in some instances they are used to avoid intervention by regulatory agencies because they refer to something that is tough to measure. Here are a few of my favorite nebulous anti-aging and beauty terms: *radiant, revitalize, rejuvenate, vibrant, glowing, beautifying, brightening* and *reduces the appearance of wrinkles*. If you see or hear any of these words or phrases, you can assume that you are entering a science-free zone.

Drink lots of water! I found this suggestion everywhere. Jennifer Lopez is reported to believe* that it will maintain the moisture of the skin and help to delay aging. Ditto Milla Jovovich. And Jennifer Aniston allegedly drinks one hundred ounces—around twelve glasses—of water per day. As she concisely summarized in a recent interview, "I drink lots of water—water, water, water." (I hope she is never far from a toilet.) One beauty-focused publication suggests that water consumption is the absolute number-one practice you should adopt for your skin, because, well, supermodels swear by it. The article goes on to declare that we should all be drinking eight to twelve glasses a day. To this end, we should *always* carry a water bottle and, to ensure regular intake, program our smartphones to remind us to drink.

Nonsense.

There are lots of reasons to drink an adequate amount of water, obviously. Your body needs fluids. But, from a skin-care perspective, the data about water's benefits are thin. Once you are properly hydrated—via coffee, tea or anything else containing H_2O—your kidneys take over. And you pee it out. The extra water does not travel to your face to make your skin look "radiant" or wrinkle free. A 2010 scientific review, for example, found "no proof for this recommendation," nor any

---

*It is worth emphasizing that I fully recognize that a publicist or a reporter may elaborate on or modify many of the comments attributed to celebs. It is hard to tell what is an actual celebrity habit or one that has simply been manufactured by the publicity industry. I interviewed a man in the movie business whose daughter once had a job that involved writing celebrity blogs and tweets.

evidence that drinking less water than recommended is harmful to your skin. The authors conclude that, while more research would help, it is likely "all a myth."

In fact, no scientific evidence exists to support one of the planet's most enduring health myths: that we all should drink eight glasses of water a day. The idea has been around for decades. Its advocates may not realize that *all* fluids, including those in fruits, vegetables, popsicles and, yes, coffee, count toward your daily water intake. You don't, as suggested by supermodels and Jennifer Aniston, need to carry around a water bottle to ensure you are always ideally hydrated. As noted in a report from the US Institute of Medicine of the National Academies, "On a daily basis, people get adequate amounts of water from normal drinking behavior … and by letting their thirst guide them."

A 2013 review of available data did find that, if you are already dieting, drinking water might help with weight loss by suppressing appetite. Having a bunch of water sloshing around in your belly may, for instance, reduce your desire to inhale a Big Mac. But the association with weight loss was quite modest and was not found among individuals who were not dieting. In general, from a health and beauty perspective, little evidence supports the idea of consuming lots of water. Drink when you are thirsty.

By the way, as part of my commitment to a celebrity-informed skin-care routine, I did try, for a short spell, to drink lots of water. I heard this advice everywhere, so I thought I should give the practice a shot to see if my face started radiating. I gave it up after a few days. I had to pee constantly! How does Jen do it? I did not notice any increase in facial vibrancy as compensation for the increased trips to the urinal. Ironically, my hands started to get dry from all the post-pee hand washing. So, for me, the impact on my skin was hardly beneficial.

Cosmetic acupuncture! As we have seen, many celebs enthusiastically embrace a range of complementary and alternative practices. In the context of beauty, cosmetic acupuncture, also called facial rejuvenation, is one of the most ubiquitous. It's a "Hot Celebrity Trend" (as proclaimed by Examiner.com), which, as one proponent declares, "celebrities have approved." It has been reported that her thrice-weekly acupuncture sessions are Sandra Bullock's secret for staying young and that she has the cost of getting needles stuck in her face built into her studio contracts. Other needle-embracing celebs include Madonna, Kim Kardashian, Angelina Jolie and the ultra-hydrated Jennifer Aniston.

The alleged benefits, as outlined by the numerous clinic websites I reviewed, include the elimination of wrinkles, a reduction in double chin and sagging jowls, brightened eyes (!), improved muscle tone, elimination of oily skin, the alleviation of acne and dark spots, and improved circulation. It is promoted as a pain-free, natural and efficacious alternative to Botox, one that will, as one website declares, bring "changes at the cellular level." Another says that results will last three to five years! So, what does the evidence say about this miracle anti-aging cure?

Nothing.

There appears to be very little research on point. I could not find even a single well-designed study that looked at the use of acupuncture to achieve the claimed cosmetic benefits. Other researchers have confirmed this dearth of good data. Given the degree to which the practice has been marketed, and the many bold and unequivocal claims made for it, you would think at least some supporting research would exist. But, as is often the case with alternative medicine, the only proofs offered are testimonials and celebrity endorsements.

Apart from the lack of evidence, several other factors encourage us to be skeptical. First, like all uses of acupuncture, it is unclear what the mechanism of action would be. How, from a scientific perspective, could needles stuck in the face make your wrinkles and double chin go away? Many of the clinicians offering this service claim it increases "energy flow"—referring, I presume, to the ancient and enormously unscientific idea that channels, or "meridians," under our skin facilitate the flow of a life force called qi (pronounced "chee"). While a fun idea, given what we know about human biology, it is patently absurd. Other, slightly more plausible, mechanisms have been suggested, such as the idea that the needles cause "micro trauma," thus promoting inflammation. But, again, no evidence supports this theory.

Second, while some studies show that acupuncture can be clinically useful for a range of conditions, this is usually in the treatment of subjectively assessed symptoms. For example, acupuncture is said to provide a degree of short-term relief from elbow, back and neck pain or post-surgery nausea. Because the assessment of benefits is subjective, however, skeptics continue to think that they can be attributed to the placebo effect. A recent commentary published in the journal *Anesthesia and Analgesia* went so far as to suggest that acupuncture is little more than "theatrical placebo." Scant evidence suggests that acupuncture can cause long-term measurable physiological changes in humans, which would be required for an acupuncture facelift to actually work. For example, research has been done on the use of acupuncture in the treatment of Bell's palsy—a relatively common disorder that causes a weakness or slight paralysis on one side of the face. Fixing this problem would require acupuncture to have a real and measurable impact in a manner not unlike what would be needed for a facelift. A rigorous and independent review of this data found inadequate evidence to draw conclusions—which is a nice way of saying no evidence indicates that it works.

Third, in the well-designed studies that have shown acupuncture to be effective, the effect size is invariably small. Being stuck with needles may, for instance, provide more pain relief than placebo, but only slightly more. So, even if we wish to be open-minded about the possible efficacy of cosmetic acupuncture, the most that can be reasonably hoped for is a small and short-term change. This kind of modest effect, which is the norm for the studies that have found acupuncture useful, is hardly the kind of demonstration that would transform, revitalize and rejuvenate your face.

Putting skepticism aside, if you find lying on your back with needles in your face relaxing (I've tried it and found the sensation odd and not terribly soothing), go for it. Finding a calm moment in life is not easy. Getting an acupuncture treatment might afford you this opportunity. Or you could just take a nap.

Coffee to kill cellulite! Coffee is a pretty miraculous beverage. It has many well-documented health benefits, including reducing the risk of various diseases. There are few, if any, reasons to avoid coffee and there may be numerous reasons to drink it. But can coffee rid your body of cellulite? Halle Berry is probably the best-known proponent of the coffee cure for this particular cosmetic conundrum. The actress regularly covers her body in coffee grounds in the belief that it will keep her skin cellulite free and, of course, radiant.

Cellulite is common. So common that it should be considered an entirely normal human trait—not something that needs treatment. About 90 percent of women—heavy, thin, tall, short—have at least some cellulite. But despite this reality, it is one of those conditions that has been cast, often by celebrities in the service of the beauty industry, as a horrid affliction that must be eradicated, at any and all costs. (The anti-cellulite industry is worth billions.) The ridiculous degree to which this natural phenomenon is viewed as a blight is highlighted by the abuse celebrities take if, God forbid, a picture reveals even a hint of it on their hides. A 2011 cover of the magazine *Star* featured the headline "Stars Lose Fight With Cellulite." Inside were "8 pages of shocking photos!" of celebrities who had attempted and failed to rid themselves of cellulite, including the endlessly embattled Britney Spears. A candid 2012 picture of Scarlett Johansson on a Hawaiian beach betrayed a posterior that was less than perfect. (In fact, by any reasonable measure of beauty, she looked great.) The photograph led to a media pile-on. One online story, which had the blunt headline "Scarlett Johansson's Cellulite In A Bikini," posted dozens of pictures of the young actress, "in case you missed how much cellulite she has now." Another story printed her picture with this simple critique: "I know, look at that cellulite. Gross."

Given the satanic status of cellulite, it is no surprise that so many women (and an increasing number of men) pour money into the anti-cellulite industry. Indeed, it seems that a large and growing anti-cellulite movement has emerged, employing a militarized rhetoric, as illustrated in the titles of numerous books and programs, such as *The 5 Keys to Kill Your Cellulite*, *Fight Cellulite Fast*, *Eat Right to Fight Cellulite!* and (no surprise) Dr. Oz's televised "Secret Weapons to Fight Cellulite." Among the weapons employed in the struggle are liposuction (which may, in fact, make cellulite worse), massage and toning machines (save your money), special diets (how could these possibly work?), supplements (ridiculous) and a whole bunch of creams. The coffee craze is just one of the many new trends, including new "shape wear" (aka girdles), which have, as noted in numerous uncritical articles, microfiber microencapsulated with the "slimming agent" caffeine. Of course, innumerable over-the-counter creams made out of coffee also exist, including one that promises to "banish cellulite by breaking down fat and draining away toxins." Remember, always be suspicious of claims that use the word "toxins"!

But despite the huge number of products, all the money invested in the area, the constant media coverage and the massive demand, very few products—including coffee-infused creams and caffeinated underwear—have evidence to support their use. As summarized in an excellent 2010 review of the literature, "The best of the currently available treatments for cellulite have, at most, shown mild improvements in the appearance of cellulite, and most of these improvements are not maintained over time." Note that this skeptical and science-informed conclusion was aimed at *the best* treatments. The less science-based and fringe approaches—such as the food-oriented home remedies that call for rubbing honey, lemon juice, cayenne pepper or apple cider vinegar on your thighs—warrant an even higher level of suspicion. The 2010 review also found that most of the existing evidence was of a poor quality and, as a result, any claimed effectiveness for a "treatment method for cellulite reduction should be regarded as speculation." A more recent review, published in 2013, came to a similar conclusion, noting that "despite the high number of treatments for cellulite reduction available on the market, only a few scientific investigations on the efficacy of these treatments have been published." Given the size of the anti-cellulite market and the vast amount of money involved, this lack of evidence is truly remarkable and fits with the BIEB problem noted above.

There are, and no doubt will continue to be, emerging, expensive treatments that appear to be somewhat more effective than all the marginal products available now. Stories and studies have, for example, documented fancy lasers that zap the connective tissue that causes the bumpy appearance of cellulite. At the current time, you can safely assume that for most therapies any promised benefit is either exaggerated, more short-term than portrayed, or out and out false. This harsh conclusion applies also to all the Halle Berry–endorsed coffee products.

Can anything actually be done about cellulite? It seems the most effective approach is old-school weight loss and exercise. But while slimming down and building muscle can't hurt, even this far-from-easy approach has limitations. It is physiologically impossible to "spot reduce" or "sculpt" your body. No matter what celebrity trainers tell the world, no exercises exist that will cause your body to lose weight or "firm" a particular body part. When it comes to cellulite treatments, start with the assumption that it doesn't work. Save your money until good independent evidence suggests long-term effectiveness.

Spa treatments and fancy facials! The spa treatment facial—that is, the application of some kind of cream made from dirt and water (aka mud), plant products or animal parts—is one of the most common and enduring of beauty traditions. In fact, when I think "exotic beauty routine," I picture a fabulously wealthy celebrity lying on a white cot in some exclusive spa with mysterious green cream on her face and cucumber slices on her eyes. It isn't hard to find well-publicized examples to support this stereotype. Angelina Jolie is said to get a treatment that uses a cream containing the eggs of baerii sturgeon. Teri Hatcher gets red-wine baths. Mila Kunis pays thousands for diamond-and-ruby facials. And Gwyneth applies snake venom to her flawless face.

While in New York doing research for the book, I decided to check out a few of the most fashionable spas in the world, the kind of place where Mila goes for her diamond-and-ruby rubdowns. For example, the Spa at Trump in SoHo offers a range of signature treatments that are infused with gemstones. One of the spa staff, a woman named Tiffany (perfect!), showed me around the facility, noting that all their products are natural and that their oils are imported from Dubai, where, apparently, the best facial oils come from. You can get a "balancing" diamond facial, because, as explained in the spa brochure, "diamonds have been used since ancient times to balance the crown chakra, providing clarity, inspiration and enlightenment." Or you can opt for the "purifying" emerald treatment, because emeralds hold the energy of the Earth. But if your face requires revitalization—and, as I have learned, revitalization is *the* goal—then you need to go with the signature ruby rub. Rubies represent "the grounding principles of the root chakra," thus making the body "invigorated and vivacious." These gem treatments cost between

$1180 and $1300, depending on the day you haul your chakra to the Trump.

Apparently, you are never too young to get balanced and revitalized. As I was getting my tour of the spa, the staff was busily preparing for some kind of big event. "It is a party for the kids in the neighborhood," the manager explained, which surprised me, because none of the usual kid-party stuff was being deployed. But that wasn't the point. I was told with complete sincerity that "the kids will learn about what happens when mom or dad come to the spa." No knowing smile accompanied the explanation. Tiffany really meant it.

By "neighborhood" I think she meant the kids who live in and around the Trump tower and by "what happens to mom and dad," she meant facials, which were to be given out free to all the kiddies. Not sure if any diamonds or rubies are involved. As I was leaving, I saw one little girl who looked to be about six years old skip off the elevator toward the spa. She was wearing a fluffy cotton bathrobe and had her blond hair pulled back in a stylish bun. *Enjoy your revitalization*, I thought. *But if your skin were any more youthful you'd be a newborn.*

I wasn't young enough to get the Trump freebie. And I could not afford to scrub precious gems on my middle-aged—though increasingly pampered—face. Also, I don't think my chakra needed gemstone-assisted aligning. But I figured I should, at least, experience a real, celebrity-worthy facial—one explicitly aimed at anti-aging and beautification. To this end, I went to another well-known spa in SoHo. It was lauded by several "reputable" sources (i.e., online celebrity and fashion blogs) as one of the most exclusive in the city. It wasn't cheap, but the prices weren't quite as steep as those at the Trump.

The friendly staff suggested that I get a facial designed especially for men—who, I was told, make up about 30 percent of the spa's clientele. My esthetician, Jolanta, did not disappoint. She met all of my preconceived spa-employee expectations. She was professional and warm and, of course, had flawless skin. She also had an exotic yet ambiguous accent that added to the calming quality of her voice. After inviting me to put on a robe and lie down on a large and exceedingly comfortable reclining chair, Jolanta went to work. Over a ninety-minute period she applied what seemed like a dozen different creams to my face, neck and shoulders. With soothing music playing quietly in the background (it wasn't Yanni—thank you, spa management—but it resided in that sonic genus), she explained the purpose of each phase of the treatment, including exfoliation, cleansing, tightening and, naturally, revitalization.

My initial impression: Awesome! I totally get it. It was one of the most relaxing experiences of my life. I didn't want it to end. Each time Jolanta finished applying one product, I silently prayed that another was to come. I left the spa feeling pleasantly light-headed and, dare I say, pretty darn centered. But does it work? Does a facial have any true and lasting benefits? Doubtful.

Once again, very little real science—or even good science-informed speculation—backs up the beautifying claims made for spa treatments. No evidence supports the use of gems or precious metals, for example. (A 2011 review of the relevant literature explicitly stated that there was no support for the use of gold.) Remember—and this can't be said often enough—celebrity testimonials are not evidence. The fact that Gwyneth, Mila or Jennifer A, L or G rave about a particular facial is, from the perspective of science, completely meaningless. And remember the BIEB! Spas and the companies that sell spa products have little incentive to sponsor research that will show a lack of efficacy.

I suspect that many people who go to spas don't really believe that rubies, for example, will revitalize their face. Nor do they believe that oils from Dubai have magical properties. And they don't think that a Gwyneth endorsement holds any scientific weight. Rather, they go to spas to experience what I experienced: ninety minutes of bliss. The vague and unverified notion that the treatments have a beautifying effect provides an excuse to indulge. It is a culturally endorsed and market-driven relaxation ritual. That said, according to one industry report, 150 million client visits to a spa were made in 2010 in the United States alone. (The industry is huge: according to one estimate, approximately 14,000 spas operate in the US, generating an annual revenue of around $10 billion.) Many of these customers are likely paying big bucks in the belief that the treatment has tangible effects. A study of the American spa industry found that while spa-goers are seeking a variety of benefits, including relaxation and escape from the hassles of life, a significant segment—a group the researchers unapologetically call "hedonists"—go to spas specifically for beauty benefits. They are paying to look better, younger and revitalized. Of course, many celebrities fall into this category. They get spa facials before red-carpet events in order to look their best.

My spa treatment felt great, but did it do anything? Was I radiating? "You've got cotton stuck to your face," said my wife. Her underwhelmed response was backed up by the before and after pictures I took while in the change room at the spa. No observable difference. I look like the same goof in both shots. The next day my face broke out in acne.

It probably seems unfair to lump all spa facials into the same no-evidence-to-support-use category. The market includes a huge variety of facial concoctions. But unless the facial cream has some pharmaceutical-grade ingredient, in which case it would need to be regulated and tested, it is not an overstatement to say that little evidence supports the use of any spa treatment, at least if you are looking for a sustainable anti-aging solution. The *only* relevant research I could find that came close to giving spa facials credibility was a small animal study that involved the application of a particular mud-pack solution to the skin of rats, and one on the potential anti-aging qualities of Iceland's famous Blue Lagoon. The former study was experimental and the latter specific to a single location and, to be frank, not terribly convincing, as it merely looked at the possible bioactive agents in the lagoon. It did not look at the actual anti-aging benefits of hanging out in the blue water—which, by the way, I have done. (No anti-aging benefits were apparent.)

Some studies highlight other, non-beauty-focused benefits of some spa therapies, such as pain relief from arthritis. But despite a good deal of digging, I could find almost no science to support the idea that a spa treatment will make your face radiant and wrinkle free. Many of the experts I spoke with said the same thing. Moreover, not one could think of a reason why a spa treatment would be helpful, at least from the standpoint of how a facial could, biologically speaking, work. For example, I spoke with Gary Fisher, a professor of molecular dermatology at the University of Michigan and director of the Photoaging and Aging Research Program. He noted that much of the over-the-counter anti-aging market—which is where most spa products fall—is "driven by marketing, pseudoscience or, in some cases, no science." I asked him specifically about the evidence for spa treatments and he confirmed that little data exist on clinical or molecular effects of, for example, spa mud-pack treatments. "People like the feel on the face, they like the experience, but there is no science to back up benefits," he concluded. So, once again, this appears to be a largely science-free zone.

In fact, some researchers and dermatologists believe that facials might do more harm than good because they can lead to the spread of bacteria (hence my post-facial acne), and can dry and, if not done carefully, damage skin. There is no medical or aesthetic reason why you need to aggressively cleanse or detoxify your skin. It should also be remembered that the formal oversight and regulation of spas and spa products is not terribly robust.

My skin-care advisor, Kirk, agrees with the negative assessment of spa facials. He was not surprised that my skin had such a bad reaction to my celebrity-worthy SoHo facial. "Basic consumer folly" was Kirk's blunt assessment of what is driving the whole area.

SO, DOES *ANYTHING* HELP YOUR SKIN?

Given what the available evidence tells us about skin care, it seems safe to conclude that we can ignore just about all the celebrity advice, testimonials and endorsements associated with anti-aging products and practices. You aren't going to get a tangible benefit from any of the gimmicks (bird poop, leeches, snails) or, for that matter, from many of the more common anti-aging practices (facials, water consumption, acupuncture). But can anything be done to slow or reverse the aging process?

Let's start with prevention. In this regard, every science-informed skin expert I talked with said the same thing. Ditto all the relevant scientific literature. There is simply no dispute about the basic steps to skin health. They aren't sexy. They aren't high-tech. And they are obvious and well known. In fact, Kirk mentioned these items within five minutes of our initial meeting. As did almost all the other dermatologists and researchers I contacted.

First, don't smoke. As I said, obvious—but not, apparently, to the massive number of celebrities who smoke tobacco and other smokable plant products (and the 1.6 billion earthlings who currently smoke). It is deeply ironic that a community so worried about aging so often engages in one of the single most aging activities. It is easy to find photos of Sandra Bullock, Katie Holmes, Julia Roberts, Jessica Alba, Ben Affleck, Ellen Degeneres, J-Lo, Daniel Radcliffe, Demi Moore, Drew Barrymore, Kate Winslet, Kate Beckinsale, Mila Kunis, Uma Thurman, Jennifer Aniston and, gasp, Gwyneth with a cigarette in hand. No amount of snail slime, acupuncture, water consumption or sheep placenta will counteract the impact of smoking. If you smoke, all other anti-aging and health-enhancing activities are inconsequential. Smoking, even a bit, won't "keep you vibrant," as Gwyneth was quoted as saying in reference to her regular weekend tobacco indulgence. Smoking *will* make you look prematurely old and wrinkled. Smokers have thinner skin and deeper wrinkles and are more prone to various skin cancers. As noted in a review on skin care published in 2012 by University of Maryland Medical Center, "Heavy smokers in their 40s often have facial wrinkles more like those of nonsmokers in their 60s." Scary.

Second, wear sunscreen. Again, obvious—but, if you believe the stats, few of us ever put the stuff on. One Canadian study, for example, found that fewer than 30 percent of those who work outside for a living wear sunscreen. One well-known dermatologist, John R. Stanley from the University of Pennsylvania, has been quoted as saying that "sun protection is the single most important thing to ensure your skin looks good for a long time. All the other things you could do to your skin are so minor compared to sun protection." Research confirms this assertion. A recent study, published in the *Annals of Internal Medicine* in 2013, followed more than nine hundred randomly selected adults for 4.5 years. They found that the skin of the group assigned to use sunscreen on a daily basis aged 24 percent less than the group that was allowed to use sunscreen on a discretionary basis. It should be noted that this benefit was observed in less than five years. Wearing it for longer would produce an even greater discrepancy between those who use sunscreen and those who don't. You should, of course, take other steps to reduce sun exposure, including wearing a hat.

Third, sleep. This one is perhaps not so obvious. But if good skin is a priority, get your Zs. A growing body of literature supports the importance of sleep for health generally. Research has found that humans are very good at picking up facial cues that indicate people are sleep deprived. A 2010 study, for example, found that people who do not get enough sleep are rated as less attractive, less healthy and (naturally) more tired compared to those who are appropriately rested. Research also hints that a lack of sleep may cause wrinkles. A 2013 study done at Case Western Reserve University School of Medicine followed sixty women and found that those who got poor-quality sleep had increased signs of aging, including fine lines, uneven pigmentation, a slackening of the skin and reduced skin elasticity. Other studies have demonstrated a strong connection between a lack of sleep and an increased risk for a range of ailments, including obesity and diabetes. Kids who go to bed late, for example, are more likely to have a high BMI. In fact, a 2010 analysis of all relevant research found that poor sleep was a "significant predictor of death." As I said, get your Zs!

Many of us aren't getting close to enough sleep. The US Centers for Disease Control (CDC) reports that approximately one third of the population averages less than six hours a night. (Adults should get between seven and nine.) That means the skin of more than forty million Americans is prematurely aging as a result of poor sleeping habits. Forget the spa. Forget the bird poop. Go to bed!

Fourth and fifth: eat a healthy diet and exercise regularly. These last two are tricky. I love this advice and, intuitively, believe it to be true. Also, it makes sense that if you are living a healthy lifestyle—and diet and exercise are critical to achieving maximum health—this will be reflected in how your skin looks. Some experts suggest that exercise increases blood flow, which, the argument goes, is good for the skin. Makes sense. Others suggest that a healthy diet provides the skin with all the necessary nutrients. This also makes sense. But I could find only a few relevant clinical studies to support these sensible suggestions. One 2010 study of more than seven hundred Japanese women found an association between the consumption of healthy fats, vegetables (green and yellow) and fewer wrinkles. A study of more than five hundred women in the UK, China and Spain found that an unhealthy lifestyle, by which they meant smoking, eating poorly, not exercising and getting too much sun, added a staggering 10.4 years to your facial age. Similarly, a 2012 study found that the consumption of olive oil and healthy diet habits were associated with reduced skin aging. Finally, research presented in 2014 by a team from McMaster University found that exercise seems to keep skin healthier. It may even help to reverse the aging process. The researchers took skin biopsies from the research participants and found that those who exercised regularly had healthier skin with more youthful characteristics than those who did not get regular exercise.

So, given the logic of this advice and the emerging evidence, I am inclined to fully embrace the diet-and-exercise prescription for good skin. Long term, a healthy lifestyle has an impact. As one Hollywood dermatologist told me, "you might be able to get away with eating crummy food in your twenties, but as we age we need to eat healthy … it shows on the face. Not sure about the science, but that is my impression and it makes sense."

SMOKE SIGNALS AND TANNING TALES

"I exercise all the time! One, two hours a day … sometimes more. Fitness is key. It depends on the part, but you need to work hard. You have no idea. Everyone [in Hollywood] is working out."

I am sitting across from a young actor on the patio of a café in West Hollywood. He is slim and ridiculously handsome—the kind of handsome that makes you hate him until you discover what a nice guy he is, and then you like him too much. While not famous, he is a working actor who knows the business well. He has appeared in Hollywood movies and on popular TV shows. He just finished playing the lead in a film shot in

Germany. He is telling me about what he must do to remain competitive in the ridiculously competitive world of acting. And while he outlines the importance of diet ("the cliché is true, the camera does put on pounds," he says) and exercise, the young, attractive, hardworking actor smokes a cigarette. He does this without any apparent recognition of the irony implicit in the behavior. No mention of some bad addiction he just can't shake. Nothing he says suggests that I might find his words and actions incongruous. And he really seems to be enjoying the damn thing. It is his second within less than an hour.

Until I started researching this book, I almost never saw young people smoking. Sometimes I catch one of my students sheepishly sneaking a smoke outside the law school. But they always look ashamed. Addiction isn't fun, their slumped frames say, especially when it is forty degrees below zero outside. But among actors, smoking seems to be the norm. I might be wrong about this. I can't find any scientific data to support my impression that almost all actors smoke. And thanks to effective anti-smoking campaigns, the media tends to avoid publishing pictures of celeb smokers. Indeed, many publicists actively work to keep the smoking habits of their clients out of the press. But my experience in Hollywood and New York sure supports the actors-smoke cliché. (As does the reliable "data" I collected from celebrity gossip websites such as IMDb, TMZ and Lainey Gossip.) I appreciate that many smoke as a means of controlling appetite. As noted, the pressure to stay slim, especially for women, is ridiculous. Still, it is odd to see—in this anti-smoking era—so many embrace the habit.

Let's set the record straight: smoking is an idiotic weight-loss strategy. In addition to the fact that there is a good chance it will kill you (as succinctly summarized by the World Health Organization, "Tobacco kills up to half of its users"), smoking is associated with eventual weight gain, insulin resistance and an unhealthy distribution of fat—among other nasty things. As noted in a 2008 review of the relevant data, over the long haul, the "data suggest that smoking may not help to control weight.... if anything, smoking (in particular, heavy smoking) seems related to weight gain." Also, unless you plan on smoking yourself into the grave, you will also put on a lot of weight when you quit (which, by the way, will likely take seven to eight attempts). A 2012 study published in the *British Medical Journal* found that, on average, people gain about eleven pounds after quitting smoking. (Note: despite the weight gain, quitting is *still* a good idea!)

What I find particularly fascinating is the dual (and always unspoken) messages emanating from the celebrity universe. Message one: be youthful and sexy. Message two: smoke. These messages are in complete contradiction. It is a contradiction for the actors trying to stay youthful and for the public who are influenced by celebrity culture.

I am not *blaming* the handsome actor for the messed-up messaging. He is caught by the paradox too. But we shouldn't underplay the influence of pop culture on smoking behavior. Research has consistently shown that the smoking behavior of celebrities can have an influence on smoking uptake. (My West Hollywood café companion looked so darn cool while inhaling that I thought about asking for a cig.) A study published in the *American Journal of Public Health*, for example, concluded, "smoking by movie stars can play an important role in encouraging female adolescents to start smoking." Other research has found that smoking in movies can lead adolescents to take up the habit. One study from 2005 found that "strong empirical evidence indicates that smoking in movies increases adolescent smoking initiation" and went on to recommend that movies with smoking should always receive an "R" rating. The situation is improving. Fewer teenagers are smoking, at least in developed nations.

The amount of smoking in movies and on TV has decreased over the past decade. Still, ample recent examples exist of popular culture's negative influence. The popular and critically revered show *Mad Men* has helped to boost the sale of cigarettes, particularly the iconic Lucky Strike brand often featured in the program. Sales of the cigarettes were twenty-three billion packs in 2007, when the show first aired. In 2012 their sales reached thirty-three billion. Apparently even drinking and smoking games are associated with the show. Participants must drink and smoke when the characters do so.

The off-the-cuff comment by Gwyneth that she has the occasional smoke because the indulgence helps her to look vibrant—something about kicking back and chilling with her friends or, as she is quoted as saying, "just the right amount of naughty"—is so ludicrous (and, from a public health perspective, so harmful) that it is hard not to be a bit angry with the actor, particularly as she has set herself up as the paragon of healthy living. It is not as if it were an incidental comment. She runs a health-and-lifestyle business and this is presented as health advice.

Of course, smoking isn't the only area where a bizarre conflict with the dominant "Look young!" message flowing from the celebrity universe is apparent. Another is in the realm of tanning and sun exposure. As noted above, absolutely every expert agrees that unprotected exposure to the sun's rays is one of the worst things you can do for your skin. Combine tanning with smoking and you are destined to look prematurely old. Guaranteed. And yet, many in the youth-obsessed world of celebrities promote the practice.

In 2013 *British Cosmopolitan* quoted Gwyneth as saying, "We're human beings and the sun is the sun—how can it be bad for you? I think we should all get sun and fresh air.... I don't think anything that is natural can be bad for you." Putting aside that absurd idea that all things natural are healthy (consider, for example, arsenic, black widow spider venom, tar sands, earthquakes, gravity pulling you toward the ground at terminal velocity), the idea that we should all be tanning is so clearly wrong that it makes you wonder what Gwyneth was thinking.

The "pro-tan" subculture—yes, this really exists, as evidenced by the many websites devoted to the maintenance of a bronze glow—loved Gwyneth's endorsement and repeated it again and again. For example, the president of a tanning advocacy group (I imagine these guys hanging in a cloud-shrouded castle with the tobacco, junk food and gambling advocates) called Smart Tan opined thus: "Hopefully Paltrow's advice will translate into other public figures taking a more sensible approach to sun care." By a "sensible approach," I don't think the Smart Tan—a term the *New England Journal of Medicine* called oxymoronic—boss was referring to avoiding sun exposure.

Virtually any science-informed expert will tell you no such thing as a healthy tan exists. This is, in fact, the opening sentence of a World Health Organization report. The American Skin Association, the Skin Cancer Foundation, Health Canada, the Canadian Cancer Society, and the UK National Health Service, among many other health-focused organizations, all have publications that repeat this axiom. Why the hostility, you might wonder? The answer is made explicit in the WHO document: "A suntan may be cosmetically desirable, but in fact it is nothing but a sign that your skin has been damaged and has attempted to protect itself."

Tanning not only ages the skin, but also is a serious health risk. Skin cancer is on the rise. It is the most common form of cancer in North America and one of most common cancer diagnoses among those younger than thirty. A 2012 study in *Mayo Clinic Proceedings* found that over the past forty years the rates of melanoma, a deadly form of skin cancer, grew by 800 percent (yep, *800*) among women and 400 percent among men. A 2010 study published in the *Archives of Dermatology* concluded that skin cancer is now an "underrecognized epidemic." And the US Centers for Disease Control has recently cautioned, "Skin cancer is an urgent public health problem, and if current trends continue, one in five Americans will get skin cancer in their lifetime." And yet, despite this grim reality, numerous studies have also found that tanning is on the rise, especially among the young. One study of US college students found that a shocking 60 percent had used a tanning booth in the last year and that 83 percent thought that having a tan was very or somewhat important.

While the developed world's affinity for a "healthy" tan, which really took off in the mid-twentieth century, has myriad sources—including a shift from the association of tanned skin with the lower class—there seems little doubt that celebrity culture has played an important role. Legend has it that the tanning fad started when fashion icon Coco Chanel was photographed with a tan she inadvertently obtained while on a Mediterranean cruise. Though this story may be apocryphal, a good deal of solid research supports the role of celebrities in promoting tanning. Nina G. Jablonski, a biological anthropologist from Penn State, has noted that tanning practices "were instigated and are maintained by celebrities, whose images are widely propagated by the media." She has also suggested that highly imitated female celebrities, such as Britney Spears and Paris Hilton, "have done much to promote both real and fake tanning, giving much impetus to booth-and-bottle, look-good-feel-good promotions at tanning establishments." Many studies support Jablonski's view. Another study, published in 2012, found that people who watch reality television beauty shows are "significantly more likely to use tanning beds and to tan outdoors than those who do not." And a 2013 study of college students found that "the glamorization of a 'healthy tan'" was a key factor in the increase in risky suntanning behaviors and negative attitudes toward sun protection.

To be fair, a few signs suggest that pop culture portrayals about tanning and the importance of sunscreen are evolving. Actors such as Victoria Beckham and Nicole Kidman now favor a more natural look. Still, the dominant pop culture message remains very pro-tan. As noted in a study from Australia that examined popular magazines, the "implicit messages about sun protection in popular Australian women's magazines contradict public health messages concerning skin cancer prevention."

By the way, just so there is no confusion, using a tanning bed is *not* a safe, or even a safer, way to tan. Some public health agencies, such as the CDC, have bluntly stated that tanning beds cause cancer. Shockingly, using a tanning bed before you're thirty-five increases your chance of getting cancer by 75 percent. It is no surprise, therefore, that the World Health Organization has classified tanning devices as carcinogenic.

The paradoxes that flow from the tension between the obsession with a youthful appearance and the aging effects of sun exposure and tanning are made all the more bizarre by the fact that research tells us that the public still equates a bronze complexion with health, vitality and youthfulness even though, from a biological perspective, it represents skin damage, decay and accelerated aging. As with so many activities, people eventually come to regret their embrace of practices done for the sole purpose of vanity. A recent study out of the UK found that many adults deeply regret sunbathing in their youth—and 40 percent blame their parents for not warning them about the long-term consequences!

After rereading the preceding rant about smoking and sun exposure, I realized two things.

First, I come off as an alarmist, self-righteous killjoy. In reality, I know that not everyone who gets a tan will get skin cancer (though the relationship between smoking and ill health is a bit more certain, verging on one-to-one). It's possible that my vehemence is a defensive response, stemming from the fact that I have, for the last five decades, done a pretty bad job of taking care of my own skin. Until I got skin-care advice from Kirk and Marie, I almost never wore sunscreen, even though I have regularly spent hours and hours doing outdoor activities, such as cycling. I have frequently burned my skin and worried little. (Burning your skin is another risk factor for skin cancer.) I have also enjoyed the "healthy tan" that I developed as summer progressed and felt that it projected a youthful energy. I was wrong. So apparently no one is immune to health myths.

Second, I have ignored one of the most important aspects of the aging story: genetics. The state of my facial pores and wrinkles likely has absolutely nothing to do with my lifelong beauty regimen (that is, the occasional use of plain soap), but is the result, at least in part, of some genetic predisposition. Recent research has shown that genetics plays an important role in how skin ages. This is one reason ethnicity is an important predictor of both skin cancer risk and how skin will age. And a big difference between males and females also exists, which is also, of course, genetic. Male skin, for example, is much thicker than female skin, thus it shows signs of aging more slowly.

Indeed, the amount of sun exposure, your smoking habits and your genes probably account for more than 90 percent of the factors that determine how your skin will age. While you can modify the first two, you can't pick your parents. Genetics is luck. And, of course, many celebrities got very, very lucky. The fact that individuals who have won the beauty-gene lottery are setting universal beauty standards is a bit like using NBA power forwards to inspire people to be tall.

REVERSING THE AGING PROCESS?

Science-informed experts agree on the basic steps to prevent premature aging. But what if the damage is already done? Or what if you simply want to look younger and reduce wrinkles? For the purpose of this analysis, I am setting aside the whole concept of aging gracefully and the problematic aspect of the widespread obsession with looking young. These are important points that deserve critical attention, but here I am interested in available evidence that tells us what, if anything, can be done to make a dramatic change in our appearance. To explore this topic, I thought it best to go to one of the epicenters of the celebrity-driven youth culture: Beverly Hills.

"I was street smart, but unfortunately the street was Rodeo Drive," Carrie Fisher famously said about the notorious California drag. And anyone who has spent even a small amount of time walking its sidewalks instantly gets the joke. It is a strange place—a mix of fashion runway, over-the-top luxury shops and Vegas-style architecture. It is an unapologetic salute to consumerism and opulence. The pedestrians on Rodeo seem to come in three discrete varieties: the tourist (distinctive features: shorts, T-shirt and sneakers); the local businessperson (tan, smartphone, expensive suit/dress and even more expensive shoes); and the species at the top of the hierarchy, the serious shopper (dark tan, big jewelry/watch, sports car/SUV and, especially if over a certain age, a surgically enhanced facade).

As I stroll the street, looking mostly like I belong squarely in the first category, I wonder if the facial appearance of this last group is the result of the abundance of anti-aging physicians—dermatologists, plastic surgeons—on the streets that run parallel to Rodeo Drive. Or is the reverse true? Is the abundance of the doctors the result of the presence of this dominant Rodeo class? A complex symbiotic relationship exists, no doubt, but I suspect it is mostly the latter. The high number of people with the financial resources to pay for their services is likely the main reason so many world-renowned anti-aging experts are clustered here.

Dr. Rhonda Rand is one of these experts. As I wait to chat with her about effective anti-aging strategies, I peruse the product posters that cover the walls of her waiting room. The advertisements all include pictures of ridiculously youthful-looking women and a range of rejuvenation promises: wrinkle reduction, skin tightening and, as offered by one poster, "youthfulness that is uniquely you."

Dr. Rand is a respected dermatologist who has practiced in Beverly Hills for almost thirty years. She trained with Kirk at Harvard and teaches at UCLA. Though the rules around patient confidentiality prevent her from mentioning or even hinting at any names, it is common knowledge that she has, like many of the physicians around the Rodeo hub, many well-known celebrity clients. Dr. Rand knows dermatology and she knows Hollywood. She and her physician colleagues are on the front line of the celebrity culture. They help to create the faces that create the broader social expectations of beauty and youth. "Everyone [in this city] wants to look young," she tells me. "For many it is an expectation, part of the job. They need to look good for the camera. It is a youth culture. And not just for actors. Writers, directors, grips … there is a lot of pressure on everyone." Given this pressure, I am curious to learn what can be done. Have any products and procedures been proven to make skin look younger and less wrinkled?

THE BIG THREE

While it is a complex process that involves many biological changes, most aging (e.g., wrinkles) results from a breakdown in the substances that give skin its structure (collagen) and strength (elastin). Also, as we age, our skin gets thinner, our oil glands become less effective and our cells don't divide as quickly. Any treatment that is going to have a measurable impact must deal with at least a few of these issues, particularly the collagen problem. Indeed, in a wonderful review written for *Archives of Dermatology* (Gary Fisher was the lead author), it was noted that the available evidence tells us that "collagen fragmentation"—a natural part of getting old but one that is accelerated by factors such as exposure to the sun (photoaging)—is the primary culprit in the aging of skin.

"What can be done?" I ask Dr. Rand. "What really works to reverse the aging process?" You will note that my inquiry focuses on undoing the damage, not on surgically altering your face. I want to know if anything exists that will modify the biological processes outlined above. And to my surprise (I went into this investigation with a deep, BIEB-informed skepticism) there are—roughly, as a few other procedures and creams could fall into these categories—three reasonable and evidence-based options.

Now, I don't want this section of the book to serve as promotion for the anti-aging industry. I am not thrilled that we live in a world where this is a rapidly growing, multibillion-dollar industry. But here goes. I will be brief.

Retinoids. "Retinoids are simply *the* gold standard," Dr. Rand tells me. "There is lots of evidence to support their use." Retinoids are a derivative of vitamin A and include a range of compounds such as retinol and retinoic acid. Many studies have shown that products, usually applied as a topical agent, that contain a sufficiently high concentration of these compounds will stimulate the growth of collagen and improve the appearance of aging skin. But, as noted in a 2011 article in *Clinical Pharmacology and Therapeutics*, while the results are objectively measurable, they "can be subtle and occur over fairly long periods of time." So while effective, retinoids (and other emerging compounds that may produce biological changes, such as products containing vitamin C) are far from a magical solution to aging skin.

Resurfacing. The next broad category of effective procedures can best be thought of as "controlled wounding," a term Gary Fisher used to describe the techniques used to ablate (i.e., remove or destroy) old skin in order to stimulate the growth of new, less wrinkled, skin. Dr. Rand referred to a radiofrequency technique, but the use of various forms of lasers is probably the most common and studied approach. As with retinoids, the data are solid. Resurfacing, as it is sometimes called, reduces wrinkles. Dr. Rand, by her own admission, had used this technique on her own neck. She looks pretty amazing. A couple of caveats should be kept in mind when considering this approach. You likely need to actually create a wound. That's how, from a biological perspective, the procedure works. So any resurfacing techniques that are minimally invasive are of more questionable cosmetic value (though some evidence indicates that aggressive microdermabrasion *may* stimulate collagen production). Also, the recovery time can be significant.

Fillers. Finally, there are all the different fillers that can be injected into your face. Initially, I had no idea that these approaches could actually cause a biological change. I thought they were simply used to fill in the wrinkles. Indeed, when Dr. Rand first mentioned this approach, she said that it is sometimes used to make the faces of hyper-thin actors look less skeletal. But studies have found that fillers, which can use collagen and hyaluronic acid, stretch the skin and, as a result, stimulate collagen production.

Other, as yet unproven, technologies to treat aging skin are emerging. Stem cell research may lead to some kind of breakthrough (clinical applications are likely years, perhaps decades, away), and a few other *possibly* beneficial antioxidants may be helpful, but, to date, I think it is fair to say that these three categories capture what's currently most effective and available. I could go into more detail about the risks associated with some of them—for example, retinoids can be hard on the skin. But the important point is that, despite the billions of dollars spent and all the noise and marketing, only a handful of effective approaches exist. Of course, these are the strategies frequently employed by celebrities in order to maintain their mugs.

BOTOX

I am sure you have been thinking, *but what about Botox?*

It works. If used properly, it works very well. It's safe. It is huge. Everyone in Hollywood uses it. Some use it way too much. You don't need to hear more from me on the subject.

OVER-THE-COUNTER = UNDER-TESTED

"Whatever it is, it should probably be prescription strength," Dr. Rand said when I told her about my new beauty routine. "In many [over-the-counter] products, the dosage is so low it doesn't do anything."

Like Gary Fisher, she is skeptical about the effectiveness of over-the-counter anti-aging products. (And, by the way, like Carrie Fisher, Rand is also fully aware of the strangeness of her locale. "It's hard, but you've got to put this stuff in perspective," she said with a laugh when asked how people should respond to the youth culture pressure flowing from Hollywood.) Rand's doubt seems entirely justified. A 2012 review of the available evidence associated with over-the-counter (OTC) topical anti-aging products found that almost no good research was available. The authors' conclusion is worth quoting at length because it does a nice job of underscoring how absurd it is that a multibillion-dollar industry, one that is purportedly based on cutting-edge science, generally has no good science to back up its promises (the BIEB is a strong social force!).

> Overall, there is a great necessity for more rigorous studies of OTC skincare products. This is especially imperative because these products comprise such a significant percentage of the enormous cosmeceutical industry. The average woman in the United States uses at least 25 products containing hundreds of ingredients on her skin daily. Very few of these OTC products, which may cost hundreds of dollars, have been subjected to rigorous controlled trials of efficacy.

Not only are many of the ingredients in OTC products unproven, but when they do (allegedly) include a potentially effective ingredient, like retinol, the dosage is so low or the form of the product so unclear that the clinical value remains questionable. Key terms are thrown around in marketing as a way to make the products seem scientifically legitimate. Also, many of the chemicals used in these products, including, for example, the antioxidant vitamin C, are relatively unstable. Maintaining the chemical in a pharmaceutically useable form is not easy: simply stuffing it in a jar won't do the trick. As noted in a 2012 paper on the use of ascorbic acid (aka vitamin C) as an anti-aging agent, "Unfortunately, it seems, many products in the market still fail even the most rudimentary [stability] analysis."

Given these realities, it is safe to assume that almost all over-the-counter products, particularly any that seem too good to be true, are probably not worth your money or time. You can ignore celebrity endorsements, no matter how enthusiastic and heartfelt. Gwyneth recently used her Goop website to endorse a sonic infusion thingy, which, to quote an evidence-free (naturally) article on the product in the *Daily Mail*, "infuse[s] the outer layers of the skin with anti-aging sea serum." This is utter nonsense, but that didn't stop Gwyneth from saying, "I've been obsessed with mine ever since I started using it. I've seen a real difference in my skin."

This leads me to an interesting paradox. When I told people about my research on celebrities and beauty, almost everyone said they knew it was all bull. I don't recall a single person who said something like "Really? I was so sure Gwyneth's sonic sea serum injector really worked. How disappointing. I want my money back!" People claim to be aware that anti-aging products won't work and that celebrity endorsements are absurd. But despite this, they keep on spending thousands of dollars on these products and using them daily. It is a huge and growing industry. Some people seem to spend money on this stuff simply because it is expensive. A well-known dermatologist, Dr. Michael Gold from Nashville, was part of a panel convened to discuss the lack of evidence and unregulated nature of the cosmeceutical industry at the annual meeting of the American Society of Cosmetic Dermatology and Aesthetic Surgery. "There is now $700 moisturizer," he observed. "There may be no difference between it and a $10 one. But people will pay $700 because it's $700."

A peculiar paradox is apparent in what we think and what we do when it comes to these items. A Canadian study published in 2010 confirmed that the main reason women buy beauty products is—no surprise here—to maintain a youthful-looking appearance. The women in the study equated looking better to general well-being. And they equated looking younger with feeling younger. But despite the fact that achieving tangible benefits was their stated goal, only 3 percent of the more than three hundred women in the study thought over-the-counter anti-aging products actually worked! As noted by the authors, "women, on one hand, questioned the effectiveness of anti-aging products (and felt they were overpriced) but, on the other hand, still purchased and used them."

Amy Muise, the lead author of the study and a social psychologist from the University of Toronto, told me she was surprised by the strength of these ironic results. "Perhaps they are not sure how effective these products are but figure it can't hurt and may help a little bit or be preventive of future aging. I think that part of the cultural ideals that looking good, beautiful, your best and looking young plays a role.... Even women who find these products gimmicky, or want to embrace natural aging, cannot escape these deeply embedded cultural norms."

Before I leave Dr. Rand's 90210 office, I ask her what she would do to improve my aging face. Is it a lost cause? She moves a bit closer, leans in and her expression immediately changes. She is no longer looking at me. She is now *examining* me. Just a few seconds later she has a verdict: she'd consider filler on my cheeks and, perhaps, some Botox between my eyebrows. Given how quickly she made this assessment, I wonder if she was deliberating on my many imperfections throughout our conversation. It must be an occupational hazard, particularly in Beverly Hills, where no expense is spared and *something* can always be done.

She offered no comment on my repulsive pore situation.

REASSESSMENT

Nine months after my visit with Dr. Rand, I show up for my dermatologist appointment to have the condition of my skin reassessed. I have been using the products provided at my visit to the skin-care clinic in Calgary relatively faithfully over the past year. I say "relatively" because it is difficult to get all the products through airport security and, as a result, I only do the full routine when I am home. Still, this is the most, by far, that I have ever done for my skin. I have exfoliated, moisturized, cleansed, decongested, tightened and protected for the better part of a year. The products used in the routine were expensive and the commitment of time considerable. So, have any measurable improvements occurred? Did all that pampering achieve anything?

Before I proceed, I must report a bit of a twist to my investigative strategy. Instead of going back to the original Calgary clinic, I decided to go to a *different* dermatologist, one who has no idea that this is an "after" test. This strategy, or so my thinking goes, will help to ensure a relatively objective assessment. If my skin has improved, it should be noticeable by any skin-care expert. I simply tell the staff at the new clinic that I am curious about the condition of my skin, which is absolutely true, and that I want to know what can be done to improve it.

The new clinic, which will remain nameless, has the identical Star Trek machine that was used to assess my skin in Calgary one year ago. The clinic staff takes pictures of my face just as the first one did. To be fair, I suppose calibration differences between the machines may be an issue. But any significant difference, one that would be visible to the outside world—which is, after all, the whole point—should be detectable.

The results? Not impressive. Compared to people of my age and ethnicity, I'm told, my skin actually got *worse* on four of the eight assessment criteria, including texture and the all-important wrinkle category.* My skin scores are about the same (within a few percentage points) on two of the criteria, including pores. The only area where a significant improvement is discernible

---

* Just so there is no confusion about how underwhelming these results are, I am being compared to a cohort of individuals of the same age. So, don't think I got worse because I aged. All the people I am being compared to aged too.

is with the amount of porphyrins on my skin, which are a by-product of bacteria. In other words, my skin is now cleaner, which is no surprise. I have been doing a lot of scrubbing!

After the dermatologist finishes reviewing my skin analysis he recommends several over-the-counter anti-aging products, at a cost of more than $500 for a six-month supply. These products and potions will dramatically improve my skin situation, or so he promises.

Thanks, but no thanks. I've heard that before. Back to ordinary soap and water.

CHAPTER 3

PAMELA ANDERSON'S BREASTS

Few would argue with the proposition that many cosmetic surgery trends have roots in celebrity culture. One could put forward a pretty convincing argument that *all* cosmetic surgery trends—big breasts, perky noses, butt implants (this is a thing)—have roots in celebrity culture, but we don't need to go that far. The point I am positing here is simply that celebrity images play a significant role in how we all, men and women, want to look and, perhaps more importantly, with our never-ending dissatisfaction with our current appearance. As I have already mentioned (and will mention again because it can't be mentioned enough when you are discussing this topic), I fully appreciate that the relationship between celebrity culture and public perceptions and desires is complex. Indeed, a huge body of academic literature addresses this issue, and I will touch on some of it below. Of course, we can't say that celebrity culture is 100 percent responsible for a particular trend: it isn't a direct causal effect. Jennifer Aniston doesn't drive to people's homes and force them to cut their hair in a certain way. Still, we know celebrity culture plays a significant role.

This comes under the heading of anecdotal evidence, but I once spent much more than I should have on a watch because

I saw David Beckham wearing it in an interview. He looked pretty darn hip. I am wearing it as I type these words, but I think I am projecting a vibe that is more mid-life-mistake than Beckham-badass. The influence that celebs have had on the mainstreaming of tattoos—again, thanks Mr. Beckham—is perhaps a better example. A number of academics have observed how celebrities have changed the public's perception of tattoos, once viewed as a blue-collar phenomenon, now widely accepted as a white-collar trend with a degree of aesthetic and cultural legitimacy. As suggested by sociologist Mary Kosut, an expert on the place of tattoos in popular culture, the "celebrity tattoo phenomenon" has "elevate[d] tattoos' cultural status." Remarkably, 21 percent of Americans now have a tattoo. For people between eighteen and twenty-five the measure is 36 percent, and for those between twenty-six and forty, Gen-Xers, it is more than 40 percent. The industry is now, thanks in large part to celebrities and increased media coverage, worth more than $2.3 billion.

I selected cosmetic surgery as an example of celebrity influence because it is a relatively extreme act (you are, after all, having someone cut into your flesh to alter your appearance). Like a tattoo, surgery isn't easy to reverse. It is a big decision that involves numerous steps, including the involvement of licensed and formally regulated health professionals who have a legal obligation to do what is in the best interest of their patients. It is not, in other words, a trivial matter for celebrity culture to impinge on the world of cosmetic surgery.

Incidentally, this discussion is not just relevant to women. In 2011, 9 percent of surgical and nonsurgical cosmetic procedures in the United States were conducted on men, according to the

American Society for Aesthetic Plastic Surgery—a 121-percent increase since 1997.

One of the fastest-growing forms of plastic surgery is called an "arm lift." This is exactly what it sounds like: surgery (often liposuction) to make your arms look slimmer. Since 2001 the popularity of this procedure in the United States has grown by 4,378 percent. Crazy. More than 15,000 people, 98 percent of them women, had this surgery performed in 2012. What caused this love affair with the upper limb? A 2012 survey by the American Society of Plastic Surgeons found increasing attention was being paid to female celebrity arms. Michele Obama has the most admired arms (41 percent) followed closely by Jennifer Aniston (29 percent). Other celebs with influential append-ages include Jessica Biel (13 percent), Kelly Ripa (13 percent) and Demi Moore (11 percent). (Wasn't Gwyneth on the list? Recount!)

And then there's Kate Middleton's nose. According to data provided by the UK plastic surgery industry, requests for the princess's nose tripled in 2012. And the royal snout seems equally popular in the US. "New York Women Rushing to Get the Kate Middleton Nose," noted a 2013 headline from the *Daily News*. "I love the shape and size of Kate Middleton's nose and just knew I had to have it," a twenty-six-year-old told the paper. For men, an increasingly large part of the cosmetic surgery market, the desired looks include Ryan Gosling's lips and Jude Law's cheeks.

Studies have found that media exposure, including TV and magazines, is associated with both an increased anxiety about aging and body dissatisfaction, two factors that contribute to decisions to get cosmetic surgery. In addition, researchers have determined that the use of cosmetic surgery by celebrities normalizes and trivializes the process, thus increasing acceptability. Other studies have found a more direct relationship between celebrities and cosmetic surgery. For example, a study published in 2011 measured the attitudes of young adults toward celebrities. The research found that feeling a connection to celebrities, particularly celebs with attractive bodies, was a strong predictor of future cosmetic surgery. The authors conclude that the "findings present compelling evidence for a strong association between celebrity worship and a willingness to undergo cosmetic surgery." Another study, published in 2009, examined the impact of TV shows that feature cosmetic surgery, including shows such as ABC's *Extreme Makeover*, Fox's *The Swan* and E!'s *Doctor 90210*. The study, which involved some two thousand college students, was definitive, but predictable: "Viewership of reality cosmetic surgery shows was significantly related to more favorable cosmetic surgery attitudes, perceived pressure to have cosmetic surgery, past attainment of a cosmetic procedure, a decreased fear of surgery, as well as overall body dissatisfaction, media internalization, and disordered eating."

It is worth noting that the impact of celebrity, and especially Hollywood culture, is global. As one Beverly Hills plastic surgeon told *The Atlantic* about his work in Dubai, "They say, 'I want a Beyoncé butt, I want a J-Lo butt, I want a Kim Kardashian butt,' and it's amazing to think the same things I'm doing here, I'm doing over there." South Korea has the highest per-capita rate of plastic surgery in the world—according to some estimates more than 20 percent of the population has gone under the knife.

With the rise in the international profile of Korean popular culture—often called K-pop—a concomitant rise in cosmetic procedures has occurred, including radical physical alterations such as jaw surgery. The most sought-after attributes are of South Korean celebrities. These include a V-shaped jaw, big eyes and a delicate nose. To get an appreciation of the preferred look, check out the dancers on the YouTube video for Psy's massive hit, "Gangnam Style." Most unsettlingly, it appears that a significant percentage of the people getting surgery in Korea are teenagers. One story on the phenomenon reported that 20 percent of one well-known surgeon's patients were under twenty and that most requested "a certain feature of K-pop stars." Korean men are also influenced by K-pop. Their goal often is to copy the softer image of boy-heroes found in manga cartoons and popular TV shows.

In 2013 the Royal College of Surgeons in the UK recommended that surgeons avoid telling patients that cosmetic surgery will make them look better. At first, this seems counterproductive, comparable to instructing perfume vendors to tell customers that their product will have no effect on their BO. But the goal of the College is to ensure that patients' expectations remain realistic. It even goes so far as to suggest that when discussing the likely outcomes of cosmetic procedures, surgeons should avoid using descriptive terms such as "nicer" or "better" and instead employ more neutral words such as "bigger" or "smaller." This policy appears to be the result of two trends: the increasing popularity of cosmetic surgery and the growing desire of many individuals to look like, or acquire a particular feature of, a celebrity.

Nichola Rumsey from the Centre for Appearance Research at the University of the West of England and a contributor to the Royal College report has noted that celebrity culture drives interest in particular looks, such as Kate Middleton's nose, Michele Obama's arms or, as we will see, Pamela Anderson's breasts. And, she suggests, patients bring these expectations with them to the surgeon's office. Rumsey says, "[The patient's] expectation is that their life is going to be more like the celebrity in question and unfortunately that's never going to happen."

David Sarwer is a psychologist at the University of Pennsylvania School of Medicine and a renowned expert on body image, particularly as it relates to cosmetic surgery. He agrees that celebrity culture has helped to create in people an "expectation disconnect," as he calls it, between their appearance and the appearance they aspire to. "It is almost like some people want to be able to order celebrity features out of a catalogue," he told me. We both were attending a conference on the social implications of cosmetic surgery. "But there is actually a very remote chance surgery will have that kind of outcome."

I had the opportunity to speak at the conference where Sarwer and I chatted. I presented a paper on the impact of celebrity culture on the popularity of certain procedures. A plastic surgeon in the audience asked me a thoughtful question that went something like this: "If we plastic surgeons are providing the patients with the kinds of procedures they want as a result of popular culture, aren't we adding to the social pressure to get the procedure?" My response: Yep. But, to be fair, the relationship is complex. Pop culture helps to create the norms and this creates desires for or adds to anxiety about particular body parts. This, in turn, may result in cosmetic surgery requests and, ultimately, actual procedures that nudge individuals closer to the desired look, thus reinforcing the instigating norm. It is, I suspect, a self-reinforcing cycle.

Obviously people have myriad reasons for getting cosmetic surgery. Not all are driven by popular culture representations of physical beauty. Many are simply striving for what they perceive to be physical normalcy (though those perceptions are likely mediated, at least in part, by celebrity images) or believe that a particular feature may be socially problematic. For many, perhaps most, cosmetic surgery is a perfectly sensible decision, the result of thoughtful reflection and appropriate clinical consultation. Indeed, there is reason to think that the majority of individuals are pleased with the results of surgery. A 2013 study from Germany, for example, followed more than five hundred first-time surgery patients. While a not insignificant number of the patients, around 12 percent, had unrealistic expectations (such as believing "all my problems will be solved" and "I'll be a completely new person"), the vast majority said they had achieved their desired goals, at least in the short term (the study lasted one year).

These results echo past studies and some of Sarwer's own research. He was lead author on a well-known 2002 study, and another in 2008, that explored the impact of cosmetic surgery on body image and well-being. The Sarwer studies found that, in general, surgery had a positive effect. "It is true, the majority are satisfied, at least within the first few years of the surgery," Sarwer tells me. But the studies also found little evidence that the surgery had a positive effect on overall body image. It seems people are happy with the specific body part that was modified—nose, breasts, etc.—but that that does not necessarily mean they are happier with their overall appearance. "Any improvement in long-term global well-being and quality of life more broadly is somewhat questionable."

For the roughly 5 to 15 percent of people undergoing cosmetic surgery because they suffer from body dysmorphic disorder—a psychological condition that causes them to obsess over a particular body part or relatively small "flaw"—research has found that cosmetic procedures do not achieve the desired result. Ninety-one percent of the patients with this condition had no improvement in their satisfaction and 5 percent actually felt less satisfied.

Sarwer also wonders about the long-term effects, especially of those decisions influenced by celebrity-mediated norms of beauty: "Patients often articulate their desires in a definitive manner. But will they feel the same way in five years about breast implants? Views change." Sarwer's comments are pertinent for two reasons. First, recent research tells us that we are terrible at predicting how we will feel in the future. In other words, we all think we know what our future selves will value and how we will think—but we are usually wrong. A study published in 2013 in the journal *Science* used data from more than nineteen thousand individuals and "found consistent evidence to indicate that people underestimate how much they will change in the future, and that doing so can lead to suboptimal decisions." We can all think of personal examples of this phenomenon. If he had had his way, the twenty-year-old me would have had "The Clash" tattooed across his back. (On second thought, that's a bad example. That still sounds pretty cool.) In the context of cosmetic surgery, the implications are obvious.

And this leads to the second reason Sarwer's caution seems sensible. Celebrity fads are inevitably, and perhaps increasingly, transient. The popularity of Kate Middleton's nose seems destined to fade, at least to some degree. But unlike other fashion trends—from high-waisted bell-bottoms to low-rider skinny jeans—a fashion fad that is the result of a surgical procedure is not easy to reverse. And any alteration that is tethered to a particular celebrity-driven look is bound to result in a degree of long-term disappointment.

It is difficult to overstate the popularity of the beach-wear-centric TV show *Baywatch*. By some estimates, at its peak, it was watched each week by more than a billion people in some 140 countries. To put that in perspective, about ten million people watched the final episode of *Breaking Bad*—one one-hundredth of the regular audience of *Baywatch*. The Guinness Book of World Records declared it the most watched program on the planet. And it produced one of the most famous individuals of all time (I'll support this claim in a moment): Pamela Anderson.

Anderson's rise to fame is well documented. It started with one of those astronomically rare "getting discovered" moments. She was attending a BC Lions football game in Vancouver when her image was projected on the stadium's screen. The crowd cheered and, just like that, Anderson's career took off. She started in commercials, did the first of several *Playboy* spreads (she holds the record for the most *Playboy* covers, at thirteen) and, soon after, landed a variety of TV roles, including the iconic part of swimsuit-wearing C.J. Parker in *Baywatch*. After *Baywatch*—Anderson was on the show from 1992 to 1997—she appeared in numerous other relatively high-profile programs.

While many of these projects had a degree of success—including the TV show *V.I.P.* (1998–2002), which she both starred in and produced, and the infamous sex tape (1998), which she also starred in and, I suppose, inadvertently produced—by the early 2000s Anderson had, I think it's fair to say, morphed into one of the first celebrities to be internationally famous for being famous. After *Baywatch*, she was famous because she was Pamela Anderson.

Just how famous was (and *is*) Anderson? In 2005 she was named the top web search term *ever*, ahead of the terms "Christmas," "NFL" and "September 11." (Christmas needs a better publicist, obviously.) One online survey has her listed as the eighty-third most famous person in human history, behind Aristotle, Ernest Hemingway and Bill Cosby. She ranks well above that other ancient philosopher, Plato, on the fame gauge. And she also ranks high on numerous other best/most/sexiest lists. The music channel *VH1*'s Top 40 Hottest Hotties of the 90s—yes, this is an official list—has her at #2, just ahead of Brad Pitt and Cindy Crawford. I appreciate that inventories like the Hottest Hotties are hardly scientifically robust data, but they demonstrate the cultural space Anderson occupies. Given her iconic status, it is no surprise that Sacha Baron Cohen picked Anderson as the object of the movie character Borat's amorous obsessions. "I loves the Pamela Andersons," Borat says, explaining his cross-country odyssey to find and wed Pammy.

Anderson's fame is also closely linked to cosmetic surgery. To put it bluntly, she has the world's most famous breast implants. No contest. No other celebrity even comes close. And at least some evidence suggests that this reality is both a significant part of her celebrity status and, for better or worse, her most socially noteworthy and measurable contribution. In 2008 the International Society of Aesthetic Surgery surveyed more than twenty thousand plastic surgeons in eighty-four countries on the influence of celebrities on patients' choices. They found that breasts and lips were the leading celebrity attributes desired by their patients, and that "the clear choice for breast look-alikes was Pamela Anderson." In addition, as noted by sociologist Anthony Elliott in a 2011 article on the impact of celebrity culture, Anderson is one of the "key representatives of the celebrity-led plastic surgery revolution." Other scholars have noted that the rise and fall of Anderson's breast size—she has had several surgeries, including augmentations and subsequent reductions—reflects and, to some degree, influences broader social tastes associated with this particular part of human anatomy.

I have always been genuinely impressed by the way Anderson manages her public image. She projects a certain charm and unpretentious likability. And it was my impression that she has been able to maximize her famous-for-being-famous status by mixing in a dash of irony and perfectly calibrated self-deprecating humor (e.g., her role in *Borat*). As a result, she hasn't attracted the same degree of public scorn as other famous-for-being-famous celebs, like Paris Hilton and Kim Kardashian. It seemed a savvy, self-aware approach. But, to my surprise, Anderson doesn't agree with me. In fact, she doesn't think she has an image that has been, in any way, manufactured or managed.

During the early stages of my research for this book, I had an odd email exchange with Pamela Anderson. I had thought of her as an ideal person to engage on the topic of beauty and celebrity culture, particularly given her relationship to cosmetic surgery and the TV show *Baywatch*, which was more about breasts and bathing suits than plot and character. While Anderson was initially keen to do an interview, I got the sense that she did not like the direction taken by the questions I sent her, some of which asked about her exercise and beauty routine, and others that explored the tension between celebrity image and reality. She was kind enough to email responses to my questions, but that was as far as the interview would go. "I will not sit down or do a phone interview with you," she told me. Since I am not an entertainment journalist, I am certain that part of the problem was my lack of interview skills. She could probably sense the presence of a fumbling amateur. Still, I feel as if I had struck a nerve. (If so, my apologies, Ms. Anderson!) To give you the gist of how things went down, here are a few snippets from our correspondence.

She set the tone thus: "I may be the worst candidate for this line of questioning.... I will be honest with you, if you are looking for the celebrity who worked hard to 'obtain a look,' keep looking." Later Anderson was more specific, stating, "I was and still am a Tom boy." And, in response to a question about whether she was aware that she was creating an iconic look: "No, just being myself—and I was working—I was playing Characters."

Perhaps she was toying with me. Perhaps she set the mode of her response to maximum tongue-in-cheek. I'll never know. But I think it only fair to take her responses at face value. And that leaves us with an intriguing paradox. The woman who has, one could forcefully argue, done more than almost any celebrity to facilitate the growth of an industry—cosmetic surgery—that is, at its core, about taking active and rather drastic steps to obtain a particular look, feels she has done little to shape her image.

She also claimed an aversion to the concept of celebrity, a point she alluded to several times. She told me, "I really do not appreciate the word 'celebrity,' it's inhumane—and unattractive—I use my position in life to do as much as I can to help animals, the environment, the oceans, children."

This comment is fascinating, particularly when viewed through the lens of Professor Rumsey's observation that some individuals may request cosmetic surgery in order to bring themselves closer to the celebrity experience. The paradoxes pile up. Anderson inspires an action, cosmetic surgery, to obtain a look that is meant to make people feel closer to a lifestyle that she, the source of their inspiration, rejects.

Years ago I had a brief encounter with Ms. Anderson. I was in the corner of an airport lounge, working while waiting for an international flight. Ms. Anderson and her small entourage sat immediately behind me. We exchanged a few words about something meaningless like the password to the Wi-Fi connection or the weather. She was pleasant and polite. She was wearing a form-fitting jumpsuit that was cut in a cleavage-friendly manner. I remember thinking, *Gosh, she is a tiny person* and *Where does one buy a form-fitting, low-cut jumpsuit?* But at no point did I think, *Now, here sits a tomboy.*

As my conversations with Anderson underscore, a ridiculously convoluted relationship exists between celebrities, body image and the actions we take to modify our looks. Anderson's career, no doubt, benefited hugely from her unique image and that image is closely associated with cosmetic surgery, even if she sees it differently. No matter what she says or thinks, her cultural impact has been significant. The image of Anderson has a life of its own. And it can pull off a form-fitting jumpsuit.

Of course, the use of cosmetic surgery by celebrities can play out in different ways, as illustrated by the experience of Mary McDonough, one of the child actors who starred in the TV show *The Waltons*. Like *Baywatch*, *The Waltons* was extremely popular (regularly rated in the top ten) and ran for a long time (from 1972 to 1981), but in almost every other respect, it was the other show's antithesis. *The Waltons*, to my knowledge, had no shots of scantily clad beachgoers. There was probably more fabric on just one of *The Waltons'* characters than it took to dress the entire cast of *Baywatch*. The show was wholesome and earnest, and while it was not usually filmed in slow motion, as was so often the case with *Baywatch*, it was slow paced.

"I love the show," McDonough tells me. "The experience was both good and bad. But I love the people. We are all still very close." McDonough played Erin, the fourth-born child of John and Olivia Walton. While on the show she had few of the terrible experiences so often associated with the life of a child actor. "*The Waltons* was a fun experience. No regrets. I have a great appreciation for the opportunity," McDonough says. But there were body-image issues and pressures. And when the show finished, the pressures intensified. Everyone seemed to think she needed to change her look in order to get new and bigger roles. And that meant, or so she was told, new and bigger breasts. "I thought that having big boobs would help my career. It was the era of *Dallas* [the popular eighties show that was big hair and big breasts]. Everyone was doing it."

But did the cosmetic procedure help McDonough? "Never changed my career," she tells me. "It didn't help. I never played a sexier role as a result of the implants." Worse, she believes that the implants had an adverse impact on her health. She had them removed in 1994.

By some estimates, almost 5 percent of women in the United States (more than five million) have breast implants. The number of procedures has increased by 39 percent from 1990 to 2010, and more than $2 billion was spent on augmentation in 2010 alone. While I could not find any data on point, the percentage of actresses—both established and aspiring—with breast implants seems likely to be much, much higher.

In September 2013, just a few months after my discussion with McDonough, the US Food and Drug Administration published a pamphlet that outlines the side effects associated with breast implants, including ruptures, deflation, scarring and pain. The pamphlet also provides a list of things anyone contemplating the procedure should consider. They should be aware, for example, that implants are not lifetime devices; they will eventually need to be removed or replaced. In addition, they should assume they will need additional surgeries, at some point, and that they will need to carefully monitor their breasts "for the rest of their lives."

"Normalization? Really? In the celebrity world it is more than just accepted now. It is absolutely expected," McDonough says in response to a question about the impact of celebrity culture. "There is a belief you almost have to do whatever it takes to succeed. Many actors and celebrities look at their bodies as a business. But, in fact, the chances of success are so rare and largely based on luck." McDonough has gone on to have a successful—and implant-free—career, playing roles on a number of well-known TV shows, including *The New Adventures of Old Christine*, *Boston Legal*, *The West Wing* and *Will & Grace*. But her experience reminds us that not only are celebrities the source of aesthetic norms but also, perhaps much more than most, they are under intense pressure to conform to those norms. They are at once perpetrators and victims.

The influence of celebrity culture on our perceptions of beauty is not always, or necessarily, negative. Celebrity status can also be used, for example, to break stereotypes and reframe the relationship between sexuality, gender and social roles. Some celebrities, such as Lady Gaga, have explicitly stated that they have a feminist agenda (admittedly, not everyone buys the claim). Other celebrities, such as actor Olivia Munn, view fame as an opportunity to chip away at the female carica-tures so dominant in popular culture. Munn, a comedian (she was a faux, and hilarious, correspondent on *The Daily Show*) and a TV and movie star (e.g., *Magic Mike*, *Ironman 2* and HBO's *The Newsroom*), has been criticized in some circles for her willingness to appear in mainstream media, such as the cover of the men's magazine *Maxim*. This and similar career decisions have certainly raised her profile, resulting, for example, in frequent appearances on those ubiquitous annual "sexiest" women lists. Munn argues that these criticisms flow from a double standard. "There's apparently no way that I can embrace my sexuality, be on the cover of a men's magazine, and also be thoughtful and smart, and know what the Pythagorean theorem is," she says.

I asked Munn, undoubtedly a rising star, what she viewed as the biggest perk of fame. I expected her to tell me something about how well she is now treated or that she loves working with terrific actors and directors. I got a much different response. "The best thing about fame is that it can be used to break down barriers," she says. "The entertainment business perpetuates stereotypes—from movies and TV to billboards and magazine covers—and it's nice when you're in a position to help perpetuate a different stereotype, one that hopefully helps change perceptions, even if it's in a very small way." This response, no doubt, is aimed at her critics.

A number of academics I interviewed hold a similar view to Munn. They note that celebrities can use their status to (I hesitate to use this word, but here I go) "empower" women and give them agency over their body and sexuality. In addition, taking ownership of an image or stereotype can change its cultural meaning (think of the evolution of "the blonde" from Marilyn Monroe to Madonna). I won't dive too deeply into this debate. But I will say that there is, no doubt, a delicate balance between producing images that may promote empowerment and those that are simply aesthetically pleasing and, as such, play to existing stereotypes. The average guy probably doesn't care about Lady Gaga's "intention" when she wears next to nothing. I simply want to highlight that this is a complex part of the story.

PORNIFICATION

"It used to be all about boobs, now it is all about the ass," Vanessa tells me. Her close friend and former co-worker, Elena, nods in agreement.* The two women—petite, curvy and quick to smile—should know. They are both adult entertainment actors or, as the rest of the world usually describes them, porn stars. Vanessa's San Fernando Valley apartment is spacious and tastefully furnished. She is an aspiring artist and her striking work hangs on the wall behind the sofa. The paintings are big, graphic and sexual. They feature naked women on their backs with their legs open, eyes locked on some unknown observer.

"I took the images from an old *Penthouse* magazine and tried to interpret them in a more beautiful and playful manner," Vanessa tells me. I immediately think of obvious metaphors for her life, but say nothing. Vanessa, who studied art in New York prior to her porn career, is returning to painting because the porn industry is dying, even here in the Valley, a locale that has long been the center of the US industry. This is happening for numerous reasons, but the biggest factor is the availability of free internet porn. If people don't need to pay, they won't.

Another challenge: more and more "porn girls," as they are called in the industry, are available and willing to do just about anything for less and less money. This flood of eager actors is due, in part, to the mainstreaming of porn and the belief that it will be a portal to conventional, Hollywood-style celebrity. One of the few studies on point, published in 2013, found that

---

* I have decided to use their real names and not their "stage names," which are of the ilk you would expect. No stereotypes broken.

a desire for money and fame are the two most common reasons people get into the porn industry.

"Many girls, young girls, get into porn because they think they are going to be famous," Vanessa says.

"It is true," Elena says. "Some new girls think they *are* famous just because they have had sex on camera a few times." Both the actors punctuate this latter comment with eye rolls and under-their-breath expletives.

"How young?" I ask.

"Eighteen," they respond in unison.

For Vanessa, the porn industry has, in the relatively recent past, been quite lucrative. She often made more than the industry standard of $1,000 per sex act (pay depends, in part, on the nature of the activity). And it has, indeed, been a ticket into the world of Hollywood's rich and famous. She is a friend—in some cases, a good friend—of many A-list celebrities. (She asks me not to name names, but it did not take much Google-ing to confirm the connections.) She tells me of matter-of-factly about wild parties at which guests are required to deposit their cell phones pre-entry. "You'd be surprised how many celebrities like to hang with porn stars," she says. I mention a big-name movie star who has a stellar reputation as a family man. "Him too," she says. "Many of my friends have partied at his house." (I am not sure if "partied" is a euphemism for a broad range of party-like activities. I don't ask. My lack of journalistic tenacity will later irritate many curious friends and family.)

Given this kind of glamour—or, at least, proximity to glamour—you can, I suppose, understand the allure of the porn star's profession. And I admit, just hearing about it prompts a certain thrill. Many of us, perhaps most, are fascinated by the party habits of celebrities, especially if they involve a throng of porn stars. And if Vanessa and Elena's descriptions are even half accurate, it sounds as though clothes are often optional and, for some odd reason, much of the partying happens in kitchens and ridiculously opulent bathrooms. But it should not be forgotten that reaching even Vanessa's level of renown is vanishingly rare, especially as porn's profitability diminishes.

Indeed, an odd paradox is unfolding in popular culture. Porn has, arguably, never had more social salience—as witnessed by the porn-star-inspired style choices ("porn chic," as it is often called) of celebs such as Miley Cyrus and Rihanna. And porn has never been more mainstream. Explicit porn to satisfy almost any taste can be accessed—and, if you believe the research on point, *is* being accessed—at any moment on a computer or, even, a smartphone. As a result, porn now appears to be a less extreme career choice than it once was. This is happening at a time when achieving fame via porn is becoming less and less likely. (I will refrain from commenting on the personal costs often associated with this career choice, including ubiquitous drug use and the exploitation of naive "newbies" who don't know what they've signed up for—two issues noted by both Vanessa and Elena.) In other words, the same forces—mostly free internet porn—that are normalizing porn and making it seem like a vehicle to fame are also making the likelihood of generating fame by way of a successful porn career less and less probable. "There just isn't as much work," Vanessa says. "And there aren't as many porn blockbusters making girls well known."

Of course, porn is also having a profound influence on more than just the fashion choices of pop stars and the career ambitions of celebrity wannabes. The current "pornsplosion," as some commentators have called it, is also having a measurable impact on notions of beauty and what is deemed erotic, as illustrated by Vanessa and Elena's observation regarding the shift in focus from the bosom to the derriere. And, at the same time, porn is having an effect on the popularity of a range of cosmetic services, including nipple tattooing (the darkening and reshaping of the areola), anal bleaching (the lightening of the area around ... well, you get the idea) and, most significantly, cosmetic genital surgery.

Over the past few years the number of procedures aimed at producing an aesthetically pleasing vagina has seen a huge increase. We live in the era of the designer vagina. Currently, thousands of these procedures are performed each year and its popularity is growing. In the United States the number of cosmetic vagina procedures is up 64 percent since 2011. A 2013 study by an industry group in the UK reported a similar rise. It also found that the average age of patients has dropped significantly over the past few years, from thirty-five to twenty-eight.

As with all forms of cosmetic surgery, the reasons patients seek it out are varied and complex. A portion of the women who get this procedure may have profound labial asymmetry or a functional impairment. But it seems hard to deny that both the growth in the practice and the particular aesthetic that is now popular—a prepubescent look that includes small labia and a flattened vulva—are a direct result of porn. A recent study published in the *International Journal of Obstetrics & Gynaecology* lends support to this speculation. The study found that women who viewed images of women with surgically altered vulvas were more likely than a control group to view modified genitalia as normal and, the authors speculate, this helps to explain why healthy women seek genital surgery.

Dr. Jennifer Blake, the chief executive officer of the Society of Obstetricians and Gynaecologists of Canada (SOGC) and a respected gynecologist, told me that she also believes that the popularity of the procedure is a direct result of the easy access to porn. Indeed, she doesn't know how else the phenomenon could have emerged. "Of course, the fashion is now little or no hair down there," she tells me. "This makes everything more visible and has added to the pressure to change how you look. But porn is a big factor." And she feels strongly that the taste for a flat and child-like vulva, which, as noted in an article in the *British Journal of General Practice* is a very recent trend, is likely to be transient. "Who knows what will be popular and viewed as erotic in the future? The aesthetic is going to change," Blake says. And that is a problem because this is a very permanent alteration. "What's gone is gone. If a problem emerges or you change your mind, you can't go back," Blake tells me.

The irreversibility of genital surgery could be problematic for a number of reasons. Many doctors worry about potential health risks. "There is absolutely no long-term data. Zero," Blake notes emphatically. The UK Royal College of Obstetricians and Gynaecologists echoed her concern when it noted that the amount of tissue removed is comparable to forms of genital mutilation, a practice associated with a number of serious, long-term complications. In fact, a 2012 article published in *The Obstetrician & Gynaecologist* suggested that there "is limited evidence to allow women to give informed consent."

A 2012 study published in the *British Medical Journal* looked at how clinics advertised this procedure. It was found that they often promise a "'youthful' vulval appearance," or a labia that is "'sleeker' or 'more appealing,'" or that the procedure will allow you to "'feel like a real woman again.'" The study concluded that "unsubstantiated claims of physical, psychological and sexual benefits were present on every website."

Some legal and ethics scholars have argued that female genital cosmetic surgery, unless done for the health of the patient, should be illegal because it exploits vulnerable women and, like female genital mutilation done for cultural and religious reasons, has many risks. Two Oxford University academics, Kelly and Foster, have argued that female genital cosmetic surgery is *already* illegal in England under the terms of the Female Genital Mutilation Act, which states that it is a criminal offence "for a person to excise, infibulate, or otherwise mutilate any part of a girl's labia minora, majora or clitoris." In other countries, such as Canada, it is also a criminal offense, unless the woman is over eighteen (which is the norm in the context of cosmetic procedures) or if the procedure is done by a medical professional in order to benefit the physical health of the woman or, to quote the relevant provision of the Criminal Code, for the purpose of "having normal reproductive functions or normal sexual appearance." Of course, many significant differences exist between female genital mutilation, often inflicted on young women without their consent and in less than ideal clinical circumstances, and female genital cosmetic surgery, performed with consent and by regulated professionals. Still, the fact that similarities exist—comparable procedures, cultural pressures that shape notions of normalcy, and unknown risks—between a universally condemned act and one that is growing in popularity and acceptance highlights the power of celebrity culture to influence social norms and motivate and normalize relatively extreme acts.

Before leaving Vanessa's apartment, I ask her about the perfect-vagina phenomenon in the context of the porn industry. What is the expectation? Given her look of befuddlement, I assume this was a stupid question with an obvious answer. "If you don't have a nice pussy, you shouldn't be in porn," she says.

IS IT WORTH IT?

One of the primary reasons that people get cosmetic surgery, particularly alterations to the face, is to look younger and more attractive. Yes, as already noted, the motivations are complex and multiple. And I don't mean to imply that getting cosmetic surgery is always a mistake. Still, few could argue with the proposition that rejuvenation and beauty enhancement are core motivations and central to the marketing of the industry. But, it turns out that, despite the dramatic nature of such procedures, cosmetic surgery's impact in both these respects can, in fact, be relatively modest.

A 2013 study published in *JAMA Facial and Plastic Surgery* sought to assess the degree to which cosmetic surgery—including face-lifts, brow lifts and eyelid surgery—made people look younger and more attractive. The researchers had people rate the age and attractiveness of patients before and after surgery. The raters were blinded, so they didn't know if they were looking at a before or after image. It turned out that the cosmetic surgery decreased the perception of age by a modest 3.1 years and, more shockingly, it had almost *no* impact on attractiveness. Other research using similar methods, such as a 2011 study on the rejuvenating effects of rhinoplasty (nose jobs), had similarly modest results.

This surprising lack of impact has been found using other approaches. For example, another study, published in 2012, looked at the value of beautification from an economic perspective. The authors, Soohyung Lee and Keunkwan Ryu, were curious to discover if cosmetic surgery was worth it, money-wise. As we will see, beautiful people make more money than their less aesthetically blessed peers, but would the costs of cosmetic surgery be offset by an increase in income? The results are consistent with the data above. The study found, in general, that "the improvement in beauty due to plastic surgery is small." And, as a result, the beauty "benefit is, on average, not large enough to justify the surgery costs." This latter conclusion considered possible increases in income from both employment and marriage. It is worth noting that a 2002 study—by the well-known economist Daniel Hamermesh—came to a similar conclusion regarding spending on cosmetics and clothing. The study found that the impact on beauty of even a large amount of spending was not huge. Most women will make back only about 15 percent of their investment in clothes and cosmetics via a beauty-boosted bump in income.

To be fair, some studies, including a 2012 analysis from Canada, found that cosmetic surgery could reduce the perception of age more significantly, particularly if a number of procedures were done. And surgery that corrects disfigurements or congenital abnormalities can have a dramatic impact. But, in general, the data on the impact of anti-aging and beauty-enhancement cosmetic surgery is underwhelming. In other words, if looking younger and more attractive is your motivation for cosmetic surgery, keep your expectations low. As the Royal College noted in their 2013 report, no one can or should promise "nicer" or "better," just different.

CHAPTER 4

WIRED BEHAVIOR

In the past few chapters I've tried to show how most beautifying activities either do not work or achieve much less than advertised. So you won't be surprised to hear that my general advice is to ignore it all. Save your money and spare yourself the psychic angst. And I stand by that conclusion.

But here is the crushing and seemingly contradictory truth: despite all my musings on the futility of most beautification activities, it cannot be denied that beauty really does matter. It matters a lot. Sure, it may only be skin deep, but the picture that skin provides to the universe has real social, economic and romantic consequences. Indeed, it matters on so many levels that it is difficult to find a realm of social interaction where looks don't have at least some impact—usually, but not always, conferring a significant benefit on those lucky enough to be beautiful. I wish the data painted a different picture. I wish I could say that the beautiful enjoy no long-term benefit. I wish I could say that we all look past appearance and measure our fellow humans solely on traits such as character, sincerity, kindness and wit. It seems deeply unfair for this not to be true. But, like it or not, we are wired up to be superficial.

This reality is hardly news. I think most of us know that looks are important. And despite a few decades' worth of academic pontification, which espoused the idea that our reverence for beauty is a social construct created by a largely male-domin-ated world, few in the academic community now doubt the social power and enduring nature of our love affair with good looks. "I sort out what it means," Daniel Hamermesh told me. "I measure its impact. Whether it is the result of genetics, evolution or how we are raised, I don't think about that stuff, but I know beauty has an impact. The research is completely unequivocal."

So, what does the research tell us? Hamermesh, one of the leading authorities on the economics of beauty, conducted one of the first studies, now considered a classic, on the social value of beauty. He remembers well the date the results of his ground-breaking study were first released, because Jay Leno used it as the basis of a monologue joke. It was 1993 and the joke was very 1993-ish. It went something like this: If attractive people earn more money, then why does Ross Perot earn more than Rob Lowe?

But despite Leno's skepticism, Hamermesh's data are pretty convincing. Attractive people make more money. Period. Worse, people with below-average looks are penalized more than the attractive are rewarded. Hamermesh and his co-author, Jeff Biddle, found that attractive people earn a premium of about 5 percent over the average looking, and homely people—as the authors bluntly categorize this cohort—are penalized by about 9 percent. These were confirmed in a 2009 study that found a similar 3 to 5 percent "plainness" penalty. The researchers also found that for attractive individuals, an increase in skill and ability is associated with an even greater increase in wages, while for those who have below-average looks, added ability may lead to *less* pay! Harsh.

Since the publication of his seminal paper, Hamermesh's work has been confirmed and refined again and again. For example, a 2005 paper found the existence of a beauty premium (this paper suggests that good-looking people earn about 10 to 15 percent more than their homelier counterparts) and broke down its source. The authors found that some of the beauty premium is likely due to factors such as the greater confidence that attractive people usually possess, but the major factor is looks. Another study takes the we-are-a-bunch-of-superficial-animals theme even further by highlighting the economic benefits of being blond. Using data from more than twelve thousand American women, the authors found that blondes receive a significant wage premium—equivalent to about an extra year of post-secondary education! Moreover, they marry men who earn about 6 percent more money than the husbands of women who lack the flaxen advantage. Whether or not blondes have more fun, they do have a bit of extra cash to pay for fun stuff.

The social advantages conferred on the gorgeous go well beyond making more money. A fascinating 2013 study, again led by Hamermesh, found that the good-looking are significantly happier and more satisfied than the plain. The large study, which includes data from all over the world, found that beauty increases happiness both directly (*Golly, it sure is terrific being attractive!*) and indirectly, as a result of factors such as greater earning power and a better education.

One of my favorite studies observed that people do not, at least when they are contestants on TV game shows and under the watchful eye of a public audience, discriminate on the basis of race or gender. But, holy cow! They sure do discriminate on looks! The study found that good-looking people are less likely to be eliminated from a show even if they perform more poorly than their average-looking fellow contestants. The authors note that this phenomenon is simply a form of taste-based discrimination and, given that contestant decisions are publicly scrutinized, stands as strong evidence of how acceptable and insidious the beauty premium is.

And it doesn't stop there. Attractive professors are perceived to be better teachers. Attractive people are regarded as more moral. Investors would rather give money to attractive men, and attractive men are 36 percent more likely to be successful. People are more willing to donate an organ to an attractive person. Good-looking students get better grades. Attractive women are more likely than plain women to marry a highly educated and prosperous man. (Interestingly, being intelligent does not seem to provide the same advantage.) Attractive people are perceived as being more intelligent and, in fact, do, on average, have a higher IQ. Beautiful people even have better, more adventurous, sex. In fact, women are more likely to have an orgasm if their partner is handsome and, in particular, symmetrical … in the face, that is.

The beauty advantage has been confirmed using a wide range of methods. For example, a 2011 study by neuroscientists from Duke University found that our brains have a shared neural pathway for the assessment of goodness and beauty. This provides biological support for the beauty-is-good stereotype (i.e., the tendency to believe good-looking individuals are more moral, etc.). The belief is, to some degree, hardwired. Specifically, the researchers found "a positive bias toward attractiveness and goodness coupled with a negative bias against unattractiveness and badness." Research also suggests this bias is very hard to overcome, even if you are aware of it. A 2014 study out of the University of Toronto found that first impressions about an individual—which are based largely on appearance—are very hard to alter. As one of the authors put it, "We judge books by their covers, and we can't help but do it" and "first impressions continue to assert themselves long after you know relevant information about a person." I could go on, but you get the idea. Beauty matters.

Given this reality, it should be no surprise that those who are deemed unattractive pay a heavy social price, and not just in terms of financial compensation. A 2013 study, for example, found that unattractive individuals are significantly more likely to be abused at work. While many studies show that good-looking kids get treated better than homely kids, this is one of the first studies to find a link between looks and workplace behavior. Sadly, looks-mediated bullying persists into adulthood. As noted by the authors, the reasons are simple: "Attractive people may be aesthetically pleasant to others, eliciting positive emotion, while unattractive people may be aesthetically unpleasant to others, eliciting negative emotion." Unattractive people have also been found to have an increased propensity toward criminal behavior, even when you control for other relevant factors, such as socioeconomic status. And, to add insult to injury, the same line of research has found that attractive people have a *reduced* propensity toward crime.

There are a few downsides to being good-looking. For example, if you find yourself convicted of murder and you are also kind of hot, you are more likely to be presumed guilty. So, before you hit the courtroom, ugly yourself up a bit. (Perhaps this explains why boyfriend-killer Jodi Arias's pre-arrest style was classic blonde bombshell and her in-court vibe leaned more toward dowdy librarian.) Also, while good-looking men are more employable than their plain-looking colleagues, some evidence suggests that attractive women don't have the same advantage—at least in the initial callback phase of the hiring process. One study found that résumés that included a picture of an attractive woman were significantly less likely to get an interview compared to résumés that had either no picture or a picture of a plain-looking woman. The authors of the study conclude, "Female jealousy of attractive women in the workplace is a primary reason for the punishment of attractive women." Ouch.

Given our established obsession with beauty—driven, in part, by celebrity culture, a point I'll return to below—you won't be surprised to hear that, despite society's efforts to fight discrimination, the effect of the beauty premium does not seem to be fading. A recent Australian study by Jeff Borland and Andrew Leigh found that over the past three decades the premium conferred on the good-looking has been constant and, in fact, has increased slightly for females as assessed by the likelihood of their being employed. While Hamermesh finds it gratifying that his early work continues to be confirmed, he is genuinely disappointed by the resilience of the beauty premium. "Why in God's name does it still exist? Ugly people can be just as smart and can reproduce just as well!" he told me. "This is a powerful force. As a source of discrimination [the economic data tell us], that is not that much different from race." As Nancy Etcoff noted in her seminal book on point, *The Survival of the Prettiest*, "We face a world where 'lookism' is one of the most pervasive but denied of prejudices." To be fair, a few anti-lookism legal actions have recently been mounted, such as the 2013 investigation into retail giant Abercrombie & Fitch for employing only good-looking people in its flagship Paris store. But, in general, our socially and biologically driven preference for attractive people is wholly unchecked. Beauty rules.

The impact of beauty extends beyond the advantages it bestows on the beautiful. It also has a remarkable influence on how we experience a range of art forms. The power of appearance on our appreciation of visual media such as movies and TV is obvious. My wife was willing to go see the zombie movie *World War Z* only because it starred the "okay-looking" Brad Pitt. (I was there mostly for the zombies.) But did you know that looks also have a huge influence on the degree to which you enjoy music? A large body of research suggests that the attractiveness of the performer affects how people respond to the performance. This isn't about stage presence or off-stage sex appeal. The fact that the 1972 Mick Jagger exudes otherworldly charisma impacts how the world appreciates *Exile on Main St.*—well, at least it does for me. This is about how people rate the *quality* of the actual musical performance. That is, the sound of the music.

The impact of looks on musical appreciation is well documented and amazingly consistent. In a recent meta-analysis, music researchers found that the appearance effect is a significant part of the listening experience. As they note, listening to music is a multisensory process. The visual component has a tangible impact on how the brain "hears" the music. And, to be clear, we aren't just talking about how girls in their preteen years judge the quality of Justin Bieber's latest single or Taylor Swift's stadium tour. This effect exists for classical musicians— including violinists, pianists and singers—as judged by highly trained music professionals. A well-known study from 1998 found that more attractive violinists received higher ratings than less attractive performers, as judged by graduate students and university music faculty members! Even people who have spent decades studying music are swayed by good looks. To be fair, some subsequent research on point has found that the power of beauty declines with increased musical exposure. But, in general, at least some of the impact endures.

The power and influence of beauty appears to be the result of a complex combination of evolutionarily determined, hardwired biological preferences and socially constructed taste. Whether nature or nurture is decisive is moot. Some of the academics I spoke to leaned toward the former explanation, others toward the latter. I have no intention of siding with one or the other as I think it is so obviously a blend of both. What was viewed as sexy and hot in medieval rural England—perhaps a full set of reason-ably healthy teeth—is obviously not the same feature that is considered sexy and hot in Hollywood today. Priorities change. Taste evolves and is not, in general, universal. While almost all researchers agree that at least some of what we find attractive (in women this means smooth skin, symmetrical features and an hourglass-ish figure; in men, it means height, and a variety of other attributes I lack) is evolutionarily imprinted on our brains, abundant evidence indicates that the local environment, whether a post-Pleistocene African savanna or a pop culture–saturated suburb, can have a tangible impact on those preferences.

A fascinating study published in 2013 in the journal *Human Nature* demonstrated the degree to which our taste in mates is the result of a complex and ever-changing nature–nurture mashup. A previous line of research found that most men find women with relatively small feet to be more attractive than women with large feet. If two women are identical except for the size of their feet, men will, on average, pick the woman with the smaller feet. An individual with a foot fetish—Quentin Tarantino, Jay Leno, Christian Slater—could probably provide a more nuanced explanation for this phenomenon, but for the purpose of this study, size was the sole (no pun intended) variable. However, the 2013 study found that admiration for little feet is not universal. The author, anthropologist Geoff Kushnick, found that approximately150 adult male members of Karo Batak, a relatively isolated agricultural community in rural Indonesia, had a "marked preference for women with large feet." When the results from Indonesia were compared with the preferences of men from all over the world, Kushnick concluded that exposure to Western culture was correlated with a preference for small feet and that preference for big feet was likely adaptive. "In the Karo Batak communities I studied," Kushnick noted, "men were overheard saying that a woman with larger feet was stronger and thus more productive in the rice fields." This study nicely highlights that even a seemingly universal and allegedly biologically determined preference can be influenced by local conditions and that the popular culture influences those preferences. Apparently, the more you see small feet in magazines and movies and on TV, the less sexy those big, strong, productive feet look.

Still, numerous other studies remind us of the biological and unconscious foundations of our preferences. There is little doubt, for instance, that traits that signal a woman's health and fertility are attractive to men. One interesting study (and a depressing one, if you are an anxiety-ridden and overworked woman) from 2013, undertaken at the University of Turku in Finland, found that stress makes women's faces less attractive to men. Specifically, the researchers found that the amount of cortisol levels in the blood (a marker for stress) is significantly and independently associated with the perceived attractiveness of a woman's face. The authors speculate that indications of stress serve as a signal of "both how healthy someone is as well as their fertility." This is, no doubt, evolution at work. Men aren't thinking, *Wow, look at those low cortisol levels ... that is seriously sexy!* For most of human history, finding a mate who was not under a lot of stress, meaning that he or she had access to food, wasn't under constant threat of being eaten by a lion, etc., was a good thing. It meant a higher chance of passing on your genes.

Another physical trait that we all find attractive, particularly in women, is even skin tone. Again, this likely relates to evolutionarily determined tastes. A study published in 2010, for example, found that men could detect even a small change in skin surface topography and that it had a direct impact on judgments of attractiveness. Another study tracked the gaze (and number of "fixations") of men as they looked at pictures of female faces. The authors found that variation of skin tone was an independent predictor of attractiveness. The more homogenous the skin, the better. This characteristic is, of course, also a visual cue of health, fertility and, most of all, youth.

THE CLOCK IS TICKING

Our society is obsessed with youth. And many researchers have cited an evolutionary foundation to this obsession. We don't want to age, at least not in appearance, and we find youthfulness sexy. Celebrity culture amplifies and reflects this obsession, as does the entire beauty and anti-aging industry—an industry that is growing rapidly as the average age of the world population nudges upward. I think this cultural fixation is obvious and axiomatic. I don't need to convince anyone of its existence, but I will say this: in the world of Hollywood image-makers, the obsession borders on insanity, particularly for women.

"I know the value of my work is more than my looks. It is confusing for me that I must look a certain way, but the industry expects that. It is … [long pause] confusing." Kyla Wise said that last word through a half smile, followed by a sigh and shoulder slump. Kyla is so unmistakably attractive that it seems absurd that the issue would concern her. But such is the entertainment industry. Just so there is no confusion, Kyla is the kind of attractive that causes strangers to pretend they are not staring—mostly men, naturally. I assume they are thinking, *Why is* that *woman sitting with* that *doofus?*

Kyla has already had a solid acting career, which started immediately after she graduated from university with a BFA in drama. She is no lightweight. She won the department's gold medal. Since then, she has had guest and recurring roles in numerous TV shows. And she has been in both independent and Hollywood movies. The work has been steady. Still, despite the enviable résumé, it is no surprise that Kyla is now both philosophical and apprehensive about her future. She is turning forty—the big 4-0—two days after our interview. I caught her on the cusp of a very big threshold, so the issues of looks and age have been weighing on her. And who can blame her? She is, after all, a female actor.

"Once [women] hit thirty, things get tough. In fact, there are few parts for women past thirty-five. There are character roles, but not many," T.W. Peacocke tells me. He is an award-winning Canadian film and TV director, so this is a trend he has witnessed firsthand. "The classic example is the movie *North by Northwest*. Cary Grant's mother is played by Jessie Royce Landis, and she is only a few years [eight, actually] older than Grant. For women, there really is a ticking clock."

Peacocke's comments may seem harsh and cynical. But, sadly, mountains of data support his cruel observations. Writer Kyle Buchanan, for example, recently published an article in which he compared the age of ten leading men and the age of the actors cast as their romantic interest. He looked at from nine to eleven movies for each of the stars. The results were unambiguous. First, the age gap in a number of cases was ridiculous. Consider, for example, Steve Carell (49) and Keira Knightley (27) in *Seeking a Friend for the End of the World*; Liam Neeson (61) and Olivia Wilde (29) in *Third Person*; and Johnny Depp (48) and Amber Heard (25) in *The Rum Diary*. More disturbing is that, for women, forty really does seem to be a major obstacle or, more accurately, a career cliff over which they tumble and disappear. Out of the 102 movies included in Buchanan's article, only eighteen had a romantic female lead over forty, and in most of those movies the male lead was substantially older, with only a handful of exceptions (for example, Richard Gere 55 and Susan Sarandon 58 in *Shall We Dance*). Indeed, around 70 percent of the female leads were thirty-five or younger. The message is clear: men can get older, but women must remain the same age.

The degree to which women are forbidden to age is highlighted by the 2013 fantasy film *Hansel and Gretel: Witch Hunters*. At the beginning of the movie the heroes are shown to be siblings of approximately the same age. These are the kids who stumble into a witch's candy house. But forty-one-year-old Jeremy Renner and twenty-six-year-old Gemma Arterton play the grown-up protagonists. Gretel must have spent a lot of time at the spa consuming anti-aging gingerbread cookies. The weirdest thing about this casting is that it elicited almost no reaction in the press. While the movie was, in general, trashed (it is one of those rare movies that is so bad it might almost be good), very few critics cried foul, or even pointed out the absurdity of the casting. I searched for rants but found only a few that pointed out the discrepancy, usually in a relatively neutral fashion. (One critic, for example, said "we can overlook" that age problem because we get to see Arterton "kicking ass.") The entertainment industry accepts this age differential as the norm. So does the public.

Many academic studies confirm this enduring age and gender bias. A 2002 study of the one hundred highest grossing films of all time found that the majority of female actors were in their twenties and thirties, while the majority of males were in their thirties and forties. Another comprehensive study of films released between 1926 and 1999 traced the negative effect getting on in years has on a woman's acting career. The authors of the study concluded "that men are allowed to age in film, and women are not. Male stars in their sixties are routinely cast as leads, even in physically demanding roles. Conversely, female stars are rarely cast as leads after they enter their forties."

Almost every corner of popular culture shares this age bias, but none more so than the fashion industry. Ashley Mears is uniquely qualified to comment on this reality—she has explored the fashion industry from the inside (she has modeled for designers such as Marc Jacobs) and is now a professor of sociology at Boston University. Mears, whose research has found that modeling is a pretty brutal and surprisingly low-paying job (a point we will return to later), tells me that "many models are recruited as young as thirteen and the average age for a high fashion model is probably twenty-three or twenty-four, but many are as young as seventeen." While Mears thinks there has been a healthy "growth in the critique and in the public awareness of this situation" she also feels that it will be hard to remedy because, as she notes, "young and thin still sells." She thinks change will have to come from the outside, that we need laws to nudge the entire fashion industry toward a more realistic portrayal of women.

It is no surprise, then, that study after study supports the tight connection between youth and beauty. A 2012 study, to cite just one example, found that attractive faces strike us as looking younger and we consider younger faces to be more attractive. Given this reality, who could blame both celebrities and the general public for scrambling to avoid a damaged dermis? A 2013 UK survey of more than two thousand women found that 91 percent were worried about the effects of aging on their appearance and a remarkable 75 percent said they were already using some kind of product to fight those effects. And women aren't the only ones who are worried. Men are an increasingly large part of the anti-aging market. A survey of more than one thousand men revealed that 60 percent regularly buy beauty products for their skin, but tend to keep it a secret. The purveyors of anti-aging products, meanwhile, have helped to make aging seem almost unnatural, as if it is an ailment. A 2012 study of 124 advertisements for anti-aging products found several key and consistent themes, including the use of scientific language to make the products seem like a "drug" that could cure the disease of aging, and, as the author put it, a twisted logic that equated youth with beauty and femininity and "older age with the absence of these qualities." The study found that the expectation that we should try to remain youthful, no matter what it takes, had been made to seem normal.

Kyla is a positive person. She loves acting and wants her career to carry on. She wants it to thrive. She tells me that she continues to take classes and audition for good parts, and has started teaching. And, by the way, she could easily pass for twenty-nine. But she is frustrated. "I constantly ask myself how do I stay competitive in a competitive business when they expect youth and a certain look? There are lots of mixed messages," Kyla says. Mixed messages? I don't think so. The message is uniform, oppressively consistent and crystal clear. Don't age.

CELEBRITY COMPARISONS

If you are a man and if you lived in a world where Homer Jay Simpson was your primary point of comparison, chances are you would feel pretty good about yourself. If you saw only Homer-esque people strolling the streets and pictured in magazines, on TV and in movies—both from Hollywood and of the ... er, homemade, erotic variety—then you would probably feel that you stacked up well compared to the rest of the universe. While you might feel compelled to stay fit and eat well for health purposes and psychological well-being, aesthetic competition probably wouldn't be a big motivator. In a beauty competition— and, as we have seen, we all seem to be in one big, never-ending pageant, where we are all simultaneously judges and compet-itors—you'd likely perform pretty well. But we men don't live in Homerworld. (Sorry, Homer.) We live in a world saturated with images of Brad Pitt, Johnny Depp, Robert Pattinson, Channing Tatum, Justin Timberlake, Tom Brady and that damn Daniel Craig (my wife's favorite). These are our comparators. Against these guys, most of us do not do so well.

For women, of course, the situation is much, much worse. It is worse in every way imaginable. Popular culture is completely drenched in images of young, thin women. In many ways, the dominant image of modern popular culture *is* young, thin women. They may not always be in the frame, but they are never far from view. One study, for example, found that 94 percent of the female characters on TV are thinner than the average woman. Ninety-eight percent of professional models are skinnier than average (no surprise) and have a BMI (somewhere between 15 and 17) that places them in the category of unhealthily under-weight. And, as noted above, older women are largely erased from or marginalized in almost all forms of popular culture. At least Brad and Johnny are around my age. For women, the pop culture comparator is almost always a female who looks like a teenager or a woman who just left her teenage years. (Gwyneth helps—she is over forty!) A Canadian study, published in 2011, determined that the idealized images of women portrayed in magazines and on TV are much more homogeneous and rigid (again, very young and very thin) than the media images of men.

While much research still needs to be done on the interplay between celebs and how we view our own physical attractiveness, one area that has received a great deal of attention is a phenomenon called social comparison. The concept is simple: We are neurologically wired and socialized to measure ourselves against other humans, whether we know it or not. We rank our success, looks and status against others. Brain imaging research, including a 2013 study done by researchers from Germany and the UK, has reinforced the idea that there is a biological underpinning to this phenomenon. Specifically, the German–UK team explored how the brain weighs "someone's attractiveness in relation to a given standard." It turns out that our brains treat beauty in the same way as other, more objectively quantifiable, traits such as height. We simply contrast one person's looks (even our own, I suspect) against the comparator's. Indeed, we use the same part of the brain to compare beauty that we use to compare height, which suggests that social comparison is hardwired even for something as socially mediated and seemingly subjective as beauty.

In general, we upward compare, particularly in the arena of looks. (As we will see later, we also frequently downward compare—often to make ourselves feel better!) Upward comparison can be inspiring, but research shows that it can also be disheartening, particularly for those who have preexisting issues with body image. Indeed, study after study has suggested that by creating an idealized standard of beauty—one that leaves us *all*, to a greater or lesser degree, wanting—celebrity culture helps to generate a social norm that is far from constructive and, I have no doubt, helps to drive the beauty industry.

Studies consistently show that media images can have an adverse (though perhaps short-term) impact on our mood and satisfaction with respect to our appearance and weight. A 2010 study of more than one hundred women found that viewing idealized images of women (i.e., fashion models and celebrities) caused a social comparison that had a negative impact on mood. Another study, published in 2013, explored the impact of media on women who were trying to eat less (which, these days, is about 25 percent of the adult population) and came to a similar result, concluding that "restrained eaters exposed to media images reported decreased weight satisfaction and increased negative mood." This kind of conclusion is typical of the research in this area. And the tendency to upward compare to an idealized image seems particularly common for women. Numerous studies have found that women are more likely than men to make an upward comparison to an idealized and unrealistic norm.

While much of the existing research has focused on women, a few studies suggest that popular culture may have an impact on men and teenage boys too—though the effect is less pronounced. For example, a 2013 study found that adolescent boys who watched music videos containing muscular and attractive singers—I am guessing they didn't subject them to any

Nickelback—"had poorer body satisfaction and poorer mood compared to boys who viewed average-looking singers."

So, comparing ourselves to hot celebrities seems to have an impact on how we think about beauty and our own appearance, a reality we have already seen in the context of cosmetic surgery. And since we do not reside in Homerworld, but in a celebrity-dominated universe, opportunities to make this comparison exist all day, every day.

HOW HOT IS YOUR PARTNER? ALAS, NOT VERY

Before we move on, it is worth noting an obvious corollary to this social comparison stuff: idealized images of celebrities also impact how people rank the beauty of others. This is at least partly because of a psychological phenomenon called the contrast effect. A classic study published in 1980 found that men rank the attractiveness and dating desirability of a woman much lower after viewing media images of attractive females. Groups of men watched the TV show *Charlie's Angels* or viewed magazine ads containing beautiful women. (Yes, in 1980, the Angels were considered beautiful, including the underappreciated Farrah Fawcett replacement Tanya Roberts.) This exposure had the predicted effect: women in the real world looked much less desirable. The authors, psychologists Douglas T. Kenrick and Sara E. Gutierres, describe the real-world ramifications of their study:

> [Imagine a man] is engrossed in an episode of a television show containing unusually beautiful females in the central role.... He is briefly introduced to a neighbor who happens

to be a female of average physical attractiveness. Our data suggest that his immediate assessment of her attractiveness and dating desirability will be lower than might otherwise be the case.

Of course, given that we live in a world where images of idealized men and women are even more ubiquitous than in 1980—*Charlie's Angels* seems quaint in comparison to, say, the flesh on display in HBO's *Spartacus*, *True Blood* or *Game of Thrones*—this contrast effect is likely operating at all times, skewing how men and women perceive the attractiveness of the "average" people we see all day long. This includes how you rate your current partner. A well-known study found that men who were asked to look at *Playboy*-type images of nude women subsequently rated their spouses as less attractive than if the comparison wasn't made.

Popular culture operates like a cruel, constantly operating dissatisfaction machine.

CHAPTER 5

BEAUTY AND/OR HEALTH?

Apparently, Christina Aguilera needed time off in 2013 from her hit TV show *The Voice* "to focus on herself," at least according to my go-to bedtime reading, *People* magazine.

I am about six months into my routine as a *People* devotee and I feel as if I have read hundreds of articles about celebrity weight loss. (In fact, according to my nonscientific calculation, 66 percent of the issues I read contained at least one article about weight loss or dieting, several of the stories featured on the cover.) They are almost always framed as admiring, good-for-her inspirational tales. (And yes, most featured female celebrities.) But this one about Aguilera stands out from the horde. First, the story has a striking presentation. The piece is built around multiple shots of Aguilera, highlighting her weight during each phase of her career. It is, I think, meant to resemble that classic image of humans evolving in stages from a small, hunched, hairy ape to an upright, posture-improved human. The point, as captured in the title, "Body Evolution," is that Christina's body has evolved from curvy to sleek.

And this leads me to the second reason this article grabbed my attention: the message reveals a cutting duplicity. One of the largest photos, taken in 2012, is an image of Aguilera at her, well, largest. Under the photo they have a quote from Aguilera that was uttered at the time the photo was taken. "I embrace my body," said the then full-figured singer. This line conveys an acceptance of the fact that humans come in all shapes and sizes. And, I am sure, that was the theme of the article when that quote was first published. But the point of the current piece is clearly that thin is best. It is a celebration of her evolution to thinness—which, according to *People*, is the result of a "fresh start"—new boyfriend, new house, revamped lifestyle, etc. As one of Aguilera's friends is quoted saying, "She is shedding the past and shedding the pounds." Evidently, "focus on herself" is a celebrity magazine euphemism for "lose lots of weight."

The idea that we all should be constantly evolving and improving—and that improving is equated almost entirely with aesthetic goals, such as weight loss, better skin, bigger boobs, perkier nose, more muscles, etc.—was a theme I came across again and again in the course of my research. "Seventy to ninety percent of women want to be thinner and something like sixty percent of men want to be more muscular," Viren Swami, a professor in the Department of Psychology at the University of Westminster, told me as we sat in his London faculty office. "If you aren't working on your appearance, you aren't normal. If you opt out [of this cultural norm] you are derided and marginalized."

Swami has spent much of his career studying the impact of popular culture on body image. He has, for example, done much of the key research on the impact of celebrity culture on trends in cosmetic surgery, finding a connection between those who follow celebs and those who get some form of cosmetic surgery. Swami says the average person is feeling increasing cultural pressure to look better and to have a particular, celebrity-defined appearance. He says that the celebrity universe invites us to ask ourselves, "Why *don't* you get cosmetic surgery? It is safe and cheap. There is this pressure to look better for yourself. The idea is that you should work on your body constantly." At one time, this fixation on body and beauty would have been looked upon as a sign of vanity and shallowness. But now, as shown by the Aguilera story, it often is presented in just the opposite fashion, as a noble and praiseworthy endeavor. Popular culture helps to normalize the relevant procedures, even relatively extreme actions such as cosmetic surgery, and the idea that working on your body is virtuous, almost righteous.

Alice Marwick, a professor of media and culture at Fordham University, agrees that our world has embraced a looks-obsessed form of self-improvement. "Making yourself better is part of the American dream, but it has morphed into the idea that you can become a better person by making your body different," she told me. I approached Marwick because of her work on contemporary celebrity culture, including a study, published in 2010, that explored how TV shows such as *The Swan* portray self-improvement. *The Swan*, which aired in 2004 on Fox, was a reality show that offered extreme makeovers, including plastic surgery, based on recommendations by a panel of experts. The whole point was that there is always a beautiful person hiding beneath that average exterior and all that was needed to reveal it was a spot of surgical modification. And striving to find that beautiful person should be viewed, Marwick discovered, as a sensible and worthwhile goal. To quote Marwick's blunt conclusion: "Television's primary answer to the moral imperative for female self-improvement is work on the body."

Studies from other scholars support Marwick's view. For example, a 2010 study of the motivations for purchasing anti-aging products found that a general acceptance of the self-improvement ethos exists and, to quote one of the study participants, "it's important for a person to take care of themselves and take pride in their looks because when you look better you feel better about yourself." Another study, published in 2013, analyzed the messages emanating from anti-aging ads, such as those featuring "older" celebrities such as Andie MacDowell and Diane Keaton. (This is "older" in the sense that their careers have survived, kind of, past the age of forty.) These women are presented as examples of successful aging, meaning, I suppose, that they don't look *too* old. The authors of this study discovered an additional twist to the self-improvement theme: the co-opting of the feminist rhetoric of empowerment. Specifically, they found that popular culture "offers the promise of self-empowerment through the use of beauty enhancement and anti-aging technologies, while also reinforcing the ideology of ageism and sexism that compels women to seek out anti-aging products in the first place."

A study of advertising for anti-aging products between 1998 and 2008 revealed a similar trend. These advertisements sell the idea that all women should strive for youth—a phenomenon the author calls a "will to youth"—by any means possible. This is presented to women as a civic duty. If you aren't trying to look younger, you are, or so the advertising implies, failing yourself and society. *That* is a wee bit of pressure. And given the size of the anti-aging industry, it is pressure that seems to work.

I appreciate that I am beginning to sound like an old-school feminist. (Not that there's anything wrong with that!) So perhaps this is a good time to point out that researchers in a variety of disciplines have commented on the strength of the compulsion to self-improve by using beauty products, going on diets and submitting to cosmetic surgery. Some have speculated that the social comparisons that drive this impulse have, at least in part, an evolutionary source. We don't want to be viewed as socially inferior—as determined through social comparison—because this would reduce the likelihood of having access to the resources needed to thrive and, in evolutionary terms, pass on our genes. And so we feel compelled to constantly "improve." (In this context "improvement" relates to a nebulous and media-facilitated notion of beauty. I do not mean to suggest that this is, in any substantive way, a true improvement.) A 2013 Portuguese study involving some 650 students, for example, explored the degree to which the need to strive—that is, to constantly improve—was associated with, among other things, anxiety, stress and the "drive for thinness." The study found that "social comparison through physical appearance with models and striving to avoid inferiority were significant predictors of the drive for thinness."

There are reasons to believe that the social comparison phenomenon is more important now than ever before. New media, including Twitter, Facebook and Instagram, allow fans to feel close to celebrities. Naturally, I follow Gwyneth on Twitter. I hear from her every once in a while—she recently told me she was hanging with fashion designer Jason Wu—but she isn't a frequent tweeter, especially compared to, say, the King of Twitter, Mr. Justin Bieber. As I write this, Bieber has around 47 million followers. (Think about that number. That is more than the population of California, Argentina, Australia or Canada.) At the time of writing, he has tweeted a remarkable 24,000 times. That is around 3.3 million characters (assuming slightly fewer than 140 per tweet)—more than *War and Peace*. While not quite Tolstoy-ian in their literary sophistication, the Bieb can produce.

By the way, Katy Perry has almost 50 million followers, more than anyone, and Lady Gaga, 41 million. Barack Obama, a man with stuff to tweet about, has a mere 40 million.

This kind of new media presence creates an artificial closeness with celebrities. It makes us feel that celebrities are regular folks who live just around the cyber corner. One day, for example, Bieber told me via his Twitter feed that it was "a great Sunday so far" and that he was attending an "amazing sermon" that made him "break down." (I pictured him hunched in a pew tweeting on his phone with tears in his eyes.) Even though the images of beauty projected by celebrity culture are as removed from reality as ever or, in fact, more so, this virtual closeness makes it easier and more natural for us all to make comparisons. "Celebrities used to be glamorous and more removed. It was fantasy. Now, through social media, they feel closer, more real and their world seems more attainable," Nancy Etcoff told me. Etcoff is a psychologist with Harvard Medical School. She agrees that social media is having an impact on how individuals feel about their looks and how they present themselves. There is now pressure to always be "camera ready," Etcoff tells me. And celebrity culture produces the images that we all, consciously or unconsciously, seek to replicate. "Even the way people pose for the camera seems to have been influenced by celebrities and new media," she says.

Ashley Mears agrees with Etcoff. She believes that new media has contributed to a growing gap between what is desired and what is attainable. "Perceptions of beauty are driven by a socially mediated desire for luxury and beauty. But it is just not obtainable," she says. "Especially since girls [models] are getting ever more slim, they are still so young, there is plastic surgery and airbrushing … all that is happening." Even the successful models Mears interviewed for her research "still feel inadequate," she says. And, increasingly, the images of these women are instantly available.

The research is still largely speculative, but some recent work supports the idea that social media is intensifying our compulsion to make social comparisons to unrealistic images. Some studies show that the more personal the relationship is between an individual and a celebrity—in academic circles, this kind of illusory social media–fueled intimacy is often called a para-social relationship—the more likely the celebrity is to have an influence on things like body image and the likelihood of getting cosmetic surgery. For example, studies have shown that having a para-social relationship with a celebrity who is "perceived as having a good body shape," to quote a relevant 2005 study by John Maltby and colleagues, "may lead to a poor body image."

Ample evidence suggests that non-celebrities appreciate the power of the images circulated through social media. A 2012 survey of facial plastic surgeons—the survey was undertaken by the American Academy of Facial Plastic and Reconstructive Surgery—found that 31 percent of the respondents saw an increase in requests for surgery as a result of social media photo sharing. Many people want to have plastic surgery in order to look good on the internet. Indeed, it was reported that some patients specifically wanted plastic surgery "due to dissatisfaction with their image as displayed on social media sites." The survey concluded that patients are "more self-aware of their looks because of social media," thus supporting both the idea that social media is intensifying the social comparison phenomenon and, as Etcoff suggested, that people want to be "camera ready." Not only are people comparing themselves to images of celebrities, they are altering their own image in order to compete in a perpetual internet beauty competition and thereby heightening the importance of and—I am guessing here, as I could not find any data directly on point—narrowing the conception of beauty. It's as if we are all in an "attractiveness arms race," an accelerating cycle of comparison and aesthetic modification that is moving us toward an attractiveness singularity that will cause the human race to be destroyed in a vast implosion of silicon, Botox, ab flexers and eternal dissatisfaction. I exaggerate. Slightly.

Of course, new media such as Twitter also serves as a forum to share ideas about social comparison. A 2013 study examined almost one thousand tweets sent before and during the *Victoria's Secret Fashion Show*. The authors found that many of the tweets demonstrated a harsh upward comparison to the fashion models. The lead author, psychologist Joan Chrisler, told me that she got the response she expected, but was "struck by the tone of some of the tweets, particularly those that mentioned self-harm." She is not kidding. Here are some of the tweets that Chrisler sent me to illustrate her point: "Eating a burrito then watching the Victoria's Secret Fashion Show then crying while vomiting while slashing my wrists with a Gillette Venus"; "VICTORIA'S

SECRET FASHION SHOW DRINKING GAME: drink every time you want to kill yourself"; and "The Victoria's Secret Fashion Show is pretty much the Super Bowl of bulimia isn't it?"

Chrisler agrees that "interacting" with celebrities through social media can create "a kind of faux intimacy," as she calls it. While she feels more robust research is needed, she worries that the trend is harmful. "When we compare ourselves to our real friends, who we know are not perfect, it might not be as stark or as painful a comparison as when we compare ourselves to our Facebook and Twitter 'friends' who look perfect in their carefully chosen photographs." And this, it seems, is exactly what happens. A study published after my exchange with Chrisler found a strong correlation between photo sharing on Facebook, body dissatisfaction and a drive for thinness among adolescent girls. Facebook increases the opportunity to "self-objectify and make physical appearance comparisons" with other girls and celebrities. It should not be forgotten that easy access to a vast quantity of images of idealized humans is a relatively recent technological development. Constantly being exposed to high-definition pictures of beautiful celebrities is, in the modern world, taken for granted. They are simply a part of our everyday experience. But just a couple of hundred years ago, the only images available of other men or women were either the people themselves, physically present, or a painting or drawing of them. For most of the population, I bet, even high-quality versions of the latter were relatively rare. So your comparators were real humans. Sure, strolling the streets of, say, Stockholm can be pretty demoralizing to the average Canadian. (I am pretty sure Sweden has some kind of cruel beauty bylaw that banishes average-looking people to a colony north of the

Arctic Circle.) But now our social comparators are rarely real. They are illusions created by pop culture.

One wonders what the future will hold. As computer-generated imagery (CGI) technology increases in sophistication, will our comparators become completely removed from reality? Will they evolve from the largely fabricated (i.e., cosmetically enhanced, airbrushed and genetically lucky celebrities) to the completely fabricated (i.e., a computer-generated image)? There are hints this could happen. In fall 2013, an incredibly lifelike computer-generated image of a ten-year-old girl named "Sweetie" was used to lure and capture more than a thousand pedophiles. The men thought the image was of a real girl, so real that they offered to pay her to perform sex acts. (Some men reportedly asked her if she had a younger sister.) The sting operation, which did not involve law enforcement officials, was conducted by the children's advocacy charity Terre des Hommes. The case is disturbing, but it serves to highlight the power of CGI. More than twenty thousand men tried to contact this nonexistent girl.

To be clear, I am *not* bashing the idea of losing weight or adopting a healthy, active lifestyle. On the contrary, losing a significant amount of weight and keeping it off is a tremendous achievement—whether or not you are a celebrity. Good for you, Christina Aguilera, Valerie Bertinelli, Jennifer

Hudson, Jonah Hill, Randy Jackson, Sharon Osborne, etc. We live in a society where approximately 60 percent of the population is overweight and about one third of those are obese. A recent study by researchers at Columbia University estimated that 18.2 percent of premature deaths in the United States are related to excessive body mass. Worldwide, nearly 2.8 million people die each year as a result of obesity and the conditions it causes. This is a serious public health issue, perhaps the defining health challenge of our generation. But the message that flows from the celebrity universe rarely has anything to do with health. The message is almost always about appearance. It is about looking great. And even when this theme is connected to the concept of health, the overriding message is that looking great will make you feel great.

Emme looks great. It is no surprise that she has *twice* been named one of *People*'s 50 Most Beautiful People in the world and was *Glamour* magazine's woman of the year in 1997. She has that beautiful-person aura: that effortless center-of-attention pull. Indeed, moments after I meet Emme—she is one of those famous individuals who have dispensed with a last name—I find myself reflecting on the beauty research referred to above. *Does Emme's great energy and confidence make her more beautiful, or did beauty give her more confidence, which, in turn, made her more beautiful?*

I am hanging out with Emme in her New York office, where she is coordinating her latest project, Emme Nation. As she shows me around, she introduces me to several enthusiastic young interns. These aren't aspiring models or designers trying to break into the fashion industry. These are university students interested in women's health and well-being. And Emme Nation is not a fashion enterprise. It isn't a clothing line. It can best be described as a healthy lifestyle forum. Emme is the world's most famous and, arguably, successful plus-size model. She is tall and looks like she could still be an elite rower, which was what she was doing when, as she tells it, she "fell into modeling." While she is still involved in the fashion world, her career focus has changed. One of Emme's current goals is to advocate for a healthy body image, a cause she is uniquely qualified to champion. She wants to nudge the fashion industry away from the "tyranny of thinness." She is, for example, working with Syracuse University's School of Design to encourage upcoming designers to have a more inclusive view of the female body. This plan includes simple, practical steps such as helping students create design mannequins that reflect the way most women are built. She doesn't want to take the glamour or excitement out of fashion. She simply wants it to be less demoralizing for the average person.

"Celebrity culture and the beauty industry is designed to make you feel bad," Emme says. And, sadly, these social forces seem to be winning. A 2011 survey of American women found a staggering 97 percent had at least one "I hate my body" thought each day and, on average, women have thirteen negative thoughts about their body daily. (This frequency, incidentally, is just slightly lower than the number of times men think about sex in a day, which is not, contrary to the urban myth, once every seven seconds.) "We create unhappiness to sell product," Emme continues, inadvertently (at least I think it is inadvertent because she doesn't dress like a Marxist) summarizing the old leftist critique of consumer culture. "We sell a type of beauty that is unattainable by 98 percent of women."

Because self-improvement is not about health or well-being, we are all caught, men included, in a bizarre health/beauty paradox. Our primary motivation for self-improvement, as sold to us by popular culture and, I think, as wired in our brains, is to achieve aesthetic changes to our body. But a combination of biological predisposition, circumstance and the ravages inflicted by time means that the vast majority of us are incapable of achieving the aesthetic ideal and, as a result, we end up discouraged and unhappy. Most worryingly, perhaps, we are dissuaded from undertaking the kind of activities that may, in the long term, have significant health and happiness benefits.

A good deal of research has been done on this dilemma. One study, published in 2013, examined more than five thousand pages of popular women's health-and-fitness magazines, including *Fitness*, *Self*, *Shape*, *Health* and *Prevention*. The researchers found, no surprise, weight loss and body shaping to be major topics, taking up more than one fifth of all content. More importantly, however, the focus of the articles was largely on appearance as opposed to health—that is, they pushed the idea that the reason to diet and exercise is to look good, not to be healthy. This was the same conclusion of a 2010 study of six years' worth of women's health magazines. In this study it was found that appearance was the dominant frame as often as health (remember, these were magazines allegedly focused on health). This study also explored how women reacted to these messages and found that after just twelve to eighteen minutes of exposure women "felt more shameful about their appearance and more motivated to exercise to improve their appearance."

The frame of the articles I read in *People* was almost always focused on looks. "Miranda's Brand-New Look!," "Hottest

Diets!," etc. Moreover, they were often associated with unscientific advice about how to lose weight. (Cleansing! Juicing!) Incidentally, the number of articles about losing weight after giving birth astounded me. Readers must love this stuff. For example, one multi-page article was entitled "Body After Baby!: How Hollywood's Hottest New Mommies Got Their Sexy Silhouettes Back." It included pictures of the women with labels indicating how fast they shed the pregnancy weight gain: Kristen Bell—"4 Months After Baby," Jenna Dewan-Tatum—"2 Months After Baby." The fact that looks are a central theme probably surprises no one: we are, as we have seen, evolutionarily wired to focus on and care about appearances. Indeed, research has consistently supported the idea that this is one of the primary motivations for people to diet and exercise. A recent study of almost three thousand people involved in the National Weight Control Registry, for instance, found that for young adults (defined as younger than thirty-five), appearance was a more significant motivator than health in the context of weight loss. Other studies have found that this is a primary reason people, particularly women, exercise. A 2008 study of nearly forty thousand university students found that 72.3 percent of the respondents were exercising in order to lose weight, and this was largely for body-image reasons. (By the way, research also consistently shows that exercise alone is *not* an effective weight-loss strategy!) Even older individuals—people at a stage in life when, you would think, they would be pretty focused on health—recognize that appearance is a stronger motivator. A study from 2002 involved in-depth interviews with women between the ages of sixty-one and ninety-two. These were not spring chickens. Even for this group, vanity ruled. "Many of the women suggest that while the health benefits of weight loss are often the stated reason for losing weight," the author notes, "the perceived appearance dividends are the key motivation behind altering one's body weight in later life."

Some of my colleagues at the University of Alberta have conducted studies showing that the lose-weight-to-look-hot stories in magazines influence people's reasons for taking up exercise. One study of 188 individuals, published in 2013, found that participants who read the "appearance-related article [were more likely to] report appearance and body tone as important reasons to exercise." The good news is that the study also found that articles that emphasized health could also have an impact on motivation. So, perhaps all is not lost.

"The problem is that compared to celebrity stories about looks, the health message is such a big yawn," says Tanya Berry, one of the authors of the study. Much of her research focuses on the impact of media on health-related behavior. She is not overly optimistic about being able to compete with celebrity culture. "The images of celebrities are just everywhere. The influence is unconscious, I think. I personally expend a great deal of effort to ignore it and I know I am still influenced. Everyone, often just for fun, talks about fitness and health in the context of celebrities. Heck, I'm curious about Brad and Angelina!" So what? If people are exercising and dieting and focusing on themselves, who cares if appearance is the primary motivation? Who cares if they are doing it because they want to look like Gwyneth, Jennifer, Selena, Brad or Channing, so long as they are doing it? This is a complicated issue. On the one hand, a body of existing research tells us how counterproductive the focus on appearance can be. A study of more than two hundred women, published in 2012, found that appearance-based motives for weight loss and exercise are associated with a range of negative outcomes, including body-image concerns. Other studies have shown that dieting for appearance, as opposed to health, is associated with binge eating and frequent (and unsuccessful) dieting. Those who are dieting to improve their looks are also less likely to be happy with their appearance than those dieting for health (admittedly, the direction of causation is unclear). They are also more likely to be stressed out by the dieting process. In other words, dieting is especially psychologically taxing when the goal is appearance and not health. And still other studies have found that those focusing on looks are less likely to stay motivated and, as a result, less likely to adopt a long-term, sustainable healthy lifestyle. Wendy Rodgers, another colleague at the University of Alberta, has studied the impact of extrinsic (e.g., exercise to look good!) versus intrinsic (e.g., I enjoy working out and it makes me feel good!) motivation in the context of physical activity. She found that, long term, people who are intrinsically motivated are more likely to keep with it.

On the other hand, some research indicates that vanity can motivate healthy behavior change. The implication is that public health advocates should simply embrace our obsession with appearance. We have seen this tactic work with anti-smoking campaigns. When people are scared by pictures that show the aesthetic damage wrought by tobacco, some of them try to quit. Other studies have found that if you want people to avoid sun exposure, messages about appearance (unsightly wrinkles) are more powerful than messages about health (dying of cancer). The effectiveness of this approach has led some health care professionals to advocate its use in other contexts, such as in the promotion of fruit and vegetable consumption (currently, fewer than a third of us eat enough). And a few studies have found that, at least over a relatively short term and in specific circumstances, being motivated by appearance can help people achieve weight-loss goals. For example, a 2009 study of patients who had gastric bypass surgery found that those who were concerned about appearance preoperatively had better weight outcomes than those who did not. As a result, the authors recommend that clinicians discuss both the health and appearance benefits of weight loss and not dismiss "an interest in improved appearance as less worthy."

While I can see the logic of leveraging looks to achieve health goals, I am skeptical about both the long-term effectiveness and social sustainability of the approach. Too many studies have found that people who are motivated by appearance are less likely to stick with a health-related behavior. Vanity might be a good hook, but research tells us that, over time, emphasizing health and the intrinsic worth of a healthy lifestyle is the better approach. As psychologists David Ingledew and David Markland have written, "[While] harnessing the desires to improve appearance and lose weight might be a powerful means of engaging individuals in exercise in the first instance, these particular motives are unlikely to sustain participation in the long term. Therefore, the well-being and enjoyment benefits of exercise should be emphasized."

I also have another problem with the do-it-for-looks strategy. This approach would seem to subtly legitimize both the *People* magazine ethos that self-improvement is about looks and the feel-bad-about-your-looks message emanating from celebrity culture generally. It invites social comparison. (A recent—at time of writing—*People* cover lauds Kate Middleton's post-baby bod. So, if you've just had a baby and don't look like Kate, get to work!) It suggests that appearance and body modification and, ya know, looking like a celeb *should* be viewed as the central goal. This kind of messaging would, I speculate, increase the rotational velocity and soul-sucking power of the celebrity-established-beauty-standard vortex.

Here is a list of just a few of the evidence-based benefits of exercise that have absolutely *nothing* to do with appearance: better sleep, better sex, better memory, better mental health, protection against dementia, protection against the adverse effects of stress, an association with a reduced suicide risk, higher grades for kids, and, of course, all the well-known benefits associated with cardiovascular health and the reduction of risk for various cancers. A similar nothing-to-do-with-looks list could be produced for the benefits of a nutritious and calorie-appropriate diet. But, as we have seen, all of these benefits, no matter how well advertised by public health educators, seem unlikely to compete successfully as a source of motivation with even one Instagram picture of Gwyneth in a Stella McCartney bikini, an image generating significant pop culture buzz as I write. In the photo, Gwyneth is leaping through the air wearing a faux snakeskin two-piece and a big gee-don't-I-look-great smile. (And, to be fair, she certainly does.) Naturally, commentary on the image consistently affirms the lifestyle-for-looks mythology. "This is what 5-day workouts during the week and a strict diet will get you!" declares Perezhilton.com. "Looks like all those juice cleanses and a strict no-carb diet has paid off for Gwyneth Paltrow," says the *Huffington Post*. If health care providers, health systems, schools, parents and public health officials don't continue to wave the health-message flag, who will? Perez? Another problem is that if we are told looks are the goal, taking shortcuts, even unhealthy shortcuts, might seem perfectly sensible.

Currently, approximately 6 percent of high school–age boys take steroids in order to build muscle mass, according to a 2012 study published in the journal *Pediatrics*. That number is astonishing on its own, but the fact that non-athletes are just as likely as athletes to use the illegal substances makes the statistic even more shocking. Clearly, kids often are taking steroids simply to achieve a particular look. This study found that steroid use in the study group is driven, not by school sports, but by other factors such as (you guessed it) "media messages and social norms of behavior more broadly." Another study, published in *Pediatrics* in 2014, found that more than 20 percent of gay teenage boys had used steroids. The authors speculated, again, that this is driven almost entirely by the desire to achieve an idealized male physique.

Another shortcut to body modification without the justification of health benefits is, naturally, cosmetic surgery, an increasingly popular practice that, as we have seen, has been linked directly to celebrity culture. A recent, rapid growth has also been seen in bariatric surgery tourism—that is, people traveling to countries to get weight-loss surgery. These are often individuals who do not want to wait for, or do not meet the clinical criteria to get, the surgery in their home country. Many of the clinics explicitly offer these services to teenagers. The fact that media portrayals of weight-loss surgery—a 2013 study by colleagues at the University of Alberta, for example, found them to be both inaccurate and overly simplistic—promotes a false sense of what the surgery can achieve, often with reference to celebrity success stories like those of Randy Jackson, Sharon Osborne, Al Roker, Roseanne Barr and Star Jones. In reality, these are potentially dangerous procedures that not infrequently lead to serious post-operative complications. And while bariatric surgery can, from a health perspective, be highly effective, it does not always lead to the expected aesthetic result.

"Television shows, popular magazines, and other popular media have probably contributed to the normalization and routinization of bariatric surgery. Celebrities who undergo bariatric surgery generate intense media coverage," Leigh Turner tells me. Turner, a professor at the Center for Bioethics and the School of Public Health, University of Minnesota, has studied the ethical issues associated with the bariatric surgery industry and is concerned about how these services are marketed. "Patients can gain access to surgical procedures that will likely be of no benefit to them and can put them at significant risk of harm," Turner says. In other words, these international services— which often do not include the long-term clinical and lifestyle support necessary to make bariatric surgery a success—are often a dangerous shortcut to nowhere.

"We need to realize that healthy and beautiful bodies don't all look the same," Emme tells me as we stroll out of her office. When you hear that sentence coming from someone like Emme, it is hard not to agree. A few weeks after our meeting, I discover the September 1997 cover of *People*. It featured a picture of Emme with a caption declaring her the world's number-one plus-size model. The headline says "Who Says Size Counts!" But the cover is dominated by a picture of a svelte Oprah—the queen of daytime TV and the shortcut, yo-yo dieting lifestyle—with a taut tummy on display. What is the take-away message of this cover? That it is fine not to meet the celebrity-driven norm of slim or that you too can (and should) be dieting like Oprah? Who says size counts? Seems like you do, *People.*

I send Emme an email to get her impressions of this high-profile doublespeak. Her succinct critique: "It truly makes me loony."

GOOD EVIDENCE?

I have tried to be careful about how I describe the research regarding the impact of celebrities and popular culture on our lives. The preceding pages contain many "mays."

The impact of popular media on human behavior is a much-debated topic. Probably the best example of the controversy has to do with the relationship between violent video games and violent behavior. In fact, despite claims to the contrary—which usually emerge in a highly politicized context and after some horrible gun-related tragedy (Sandy Hook, Columbine, the massacre in Norway, etc.)—very little good evidence supports the idea that video games increase real-world violence. As one media researcher told *Time* magazine shortly after the Sandy Hook murders, "There is no good evidence that video games or other media contributes, even in a small way, to mass homicides or any other violence among youth."

In the realm of beauty the conventional academic wisdom is that celebrity culture is pretty evil, at least in the context of body image. Literally hundreds of studies have been done on the subject, and almost all of them seem to conclude that the idealized images of men and women stimulate dissatisfaction, shame and unhappiness. A 2010 report by the American Psychological Association suggested that the "sexualization and objectification undermine confidence in and comfort with one's own body, leading to a host of negative emotional consequences, such as shame, anxiety, and even self-disgust." But despite such seemingly authoritative statements by respected professional organizations, we can't really say, definitively, that media portrayals of thin and beautiful women have, at the population level, a negative long-term impact on body image. We need to be careful about casting celebrity culture as a malevolent force that is singlehandedly twisting how we perceive our own bodies. In fact, it is very difficult to study so complex a phenomenon. To cite just one methodological challenge, laboratory experiments (e.g., showing people pictures of thin women and measuring their response) occur in a controlled, artificial environment. In addition, research has shown that the impact of idealized media images differs depending on the characteristics of the observer. For example, one study, published in 2010, found that the weight of the women seeing the images had a significant impact on the nature of the social comparison response. We need to be careful about generalizing results from these studies. They don't necessarily show how we really respond, day to day, to media images.

Among the many other factors that can impact body image are genetics and peer pressure. The latter seems particularly important. A 2013 study of 237 girls between the ages of ten and seventeen found that peer pressure and not media exposure to thin beautiful women influenced negative views about body image. Another study, published in 2012, found that identical twins are more likely to have similar views on thinness and beauty as compared to fraternal twins. This suggests that genes play a role in how people internalize the thin ideal. Put another way, genes may cause some people, but not others, to think, as the lead author, Jessica Suisman, is quoted as saying, "I wish I looked more like the women I see in the media and magazines."

I am, at heart, a skeptic. And I am particularly suspicious of studies that try to explain tremendously complicated human behavior—such as perceptions of self, dieting, exercising, etc.—based on a relatively limited method (e.g., responses to surveys, laboratory-administered questionnaires, etc.). We should also take care to not cast the public as "naive passive receptacles of celebrity advice," as one of the scholars I interviewed put it. Most people know about the ongoing criticism of celebrity culture and its impact on body image. This knowledge likely helps to ameliorate both the interpretation and impact of idealized images.

Christopher Ferguson, professor of psychology at Stetson University, is critical of the tendency to overstate or oversimplify the impact of media on human behavior. And Ferguson does not shy away from controversy. Recently, he cast his perceptive eye over all the studies that claim that media portrayals of thin, beautiful women impact body image. His 2013 meta-analysis of more than two hundred relevant studies concluded that while media likely has an impact on some—such as those with pre-existing body dissatisfaction issues—the existing data are far from conclusive. "We all like to wag our finger at popular culture," he tells me. "It is easy to be sanctimonious, but the research is not really very convincing. In reality the impact of media is likely complicated and subtle. But [many scholars] don't let this fact get in the way of a good story. So they just repeat it like it is true." And he believes the story that is repeated that celebrity culture is ruining kids' lives.

Of course, not everyone agrees with Ferguson. A similar meta-analysis—albeit somewhat smaller—was published in 2008 and it came to the exact opposite result, its authors concluding that while the effects were moderate, "the findings support the notion that exposure to media images depicting the thin-ideal body is related to body image concerns for women."

Regardless of whom you agree with, Ferguson reminds us that we should avoid over-interpreting what the data actually say. We need to be wary of grand statements about causation and to not allow moral revulsion to twist how the research is done and what the data actually say. We need to be sure that any policy response to the body-image issue is appropriately informed by reliable and rigorously done research. Long term, we need more research—particularly, I think, work that considers the impact of social media. So, this is a call for both caution and hard work.

CUTTING THROUGH THE CONFUSION

With that big caveat behind us, allow me to provide a few broad conclusions that tie together some of the central, evidence-based themes from this section of the book. They are obvious and simple, but that is, in part, the whole point. Celebrity culture spews out such a vast amount of pseudoscientific noise that a bit of science-informed clarity is desperately needed. Numerous studies have confirmed that, despite the obvious wronghead-edness of so much of the extant beauty and health advice, people remain thoroughly confused about what actually works. Moreover, in an era when obesity has emerged as one of the biggest public health concerns, and when issues associated with body image—including some eating disorders—appear to be on the rise, celebrity culture emphasizes precisely the wrong solutions. Instead of embracing a healthy, sustainable lifestyle that focuses on long-term well-being, celebrity culture focuses on and promotes short-term aesthetic goals that are, for 99 percent of the population, impossible to achieve.

Weight-loss and diet gimmicks never work and are rarely supported by actual science. This may seem an overstatement, but both history (can you name just *one* diet fad that has panned out, long term?) and the best available research support it. And don't be fooled by the celebrity status of the endorsers, the medical credentials of the inventors or the pseudoscientific jargon that so often accompanies the claims. The best diet is the simple, balanced diet we have known about for decades.

All novel, apparently simple solutions to vague health problems are likely bogus. Alas, the human body is complex. It is rare that we can "fix" an ailment or condition through the use of one novel, "breakthrough" intervention. Be suspicious of all simple (and scientifically unsubstantiated) diagnostic tests and quick-fix solutions (vitamins, supplements, special diets, etc.), particularly when they are aimed at relatively amorphous and subjectively assessed problems (anxiety, fatigue, stress, etc.).

You don't need to detox, cleanse, juice, hyper-hydrate, supplement, etc. This one is easy. There is simply no good evidence for any of these health trends, and for some—like extreme detoxes, high doses of vitamins and colon cleanses—the evidence tells us they can be harmful. In fact, if some new health trend emerges, no matter how enticing and logical it may seem, I can almost guarantee it will lack solid science. These alternative approaches to nutrition never work. So, start with that assumption and you will likely be correct 99.9 percent of the time.

Very little reliable science can be seen to support many of the claims that flow from the beauty and anti-aging industry. Given the size of this industry, I was astounded by the lack of good, independent research. The beauty industry efficacy bias— BIEB—really does dominate this world. You can disregard almost everything that flows from this industry. Save your money. Few products and procedures will have a dramatic impact. Even in the context of cosmetic surgery—which can, obviously, result in significant physical changes—the impact, both aesthetically and psychologically, is likely to be more modest than expected.

Celebrity culture encourages a range of unhealthy behavior. Smoking, sunbathing, extreme diets, ingestion of unnecessary vitamins and potentially ill-advised cosmetic surgery are just a few of the examples that fall into this category. I don't think celebrities do this on purpose. As the experiences of people like Kyla Wise and Mary McDonough demonstrate, celebrities are subject to the same twisting forces about beauty and health that afflict the rest of us. Arguably, they are more vulnerable. This is a systemic phenomenon, not some celebrity-driven conspiracy. But the evidence tells us that, whether or not we know it, celebrity culture has an impact.

Celebrity culture helps to set unrealistic beauty norms and makes us feel bad about ourselves and our looks. While the data on the long-term impact of celebrity culture in some domains may still be iffy, the body of evidence supports the spirit of this proposition, particularly over the short term and for individuals who are already at risk. Indeed, we are likely biologically wired and socially encouraged to constantly compare ourselves to other humans. This, in our media-saturated world, often means the ridiculously attractive images of celebrities. And new media tools, such as Facebook, Twitter and Instagram, increase both the power and frequency of such comparisons. But we are comparing ourselves to illusions. This does little to contribute to our day-to-day happiness.

Celebrity culture encourages uncritical, magical thinking. One of most destructive and worrisome aspects of celebrity culture's grip on society is that it seems to facilitate a pseudoscientific approach to health and beauty. An endless parade of celebrities either peddle scientifically unsupportable ideas or, through their actions, images and statements, endorse pseudoscientific products and approaches to health and beauty. All this noise is often accompanied by an authoritative rhetoric— as we saw in our examination of Gwyneth's cleanse. But rarely is any real science involved. Testimonials and anecdotes are *not* evidence. In fact, one of the essential functions of the scientific method is to cut through the bias created by personal perceptions and the persuasive force of anecdotes. When reviewing the claims associated with new health and beauty products, we must look for good, supporting data.

THE SCIENCE-INFORMED SIX

Celebrity culture is such a powerful and pervasive force that it likely has an impact on our perceptions and beliefs even when we don't recognize it. I have had numerous gluten-free, juicing, cleansed, detoxified friends and acquaintances tell me, without a hint of irony, some version of this: "Only an idiot would listen to celebrities." But the influence is subtle and hard to ignore. Celebrity culture leverages our biologically predetermined love affair with beauty, helping to perpetuate an aesthetic angst that can never be resolved, especially by the useless products and advice that flow from the celebrity maw. We should constantly remind ourselves of the existence of these cultural forces and biological predispositions. Perhaps say a little mantra: *We should not let celebrity lies defy the science-informed six.* (Sure, I'm not Jay-Z or Eminem ... or, even, Vanilla Ice, but it works.) From a health perspective, these six steps are well known and time tested:

1. Don't smoke.
2. Stay active, exercise regularly and include some vigorous activities.
3. Eat a balanced and calorie-appropriate diet that includes lots of fruits and vegetables, whole grains, lean protein, etc.
4. Maintain a healthy weight (tough, I know).
5. Wear sunscreen.
6. Get an appropriate amount of sleep (which, for most, is between seven and nine hours a night).

That is it. Everything else is either total baloney or of such marginal value when compared to the impact of these actions as to be nearly irrelevant. For example, if you smoke or don't exercise, worrying about eating organic food is like Wile E. Coyote using that tiny, broken umbrella to minimize the effects of a house-sized boulder falling on his head.

Celebrity culture, at best, is selling us a tiny, broken umbrella.

PART II

THE ILLUSION THAT YOU TOO CAN BE A CELEBRITY

CHAPTER 6

DREAMS OF FAME AND FORTUNE

"This is such a great album!" I declare to no one in particular.

This is my reflexive, near-Pavlovian, know-it-all response to hearing the opening bars of "Wouldn't It Be Nice," the first song on the Beach Boys'—or, if we are being honest, Brian Wilson's—remarkable *Pet Sounds*.

I am standing at the counter in a Paris bookshop with my teenage son, Adam. The album is playing over the store sound system. Adam has been subjected to a lifetime of my music-related pontifications, so all I get in response is a raised eyebrow and a half smile that tells me, "Yep, Dad, I know, you like this album. And, by the way, you are kind of embarrassing."

But someone else is listening. "This *is* a great album," the cashier says in accent-free English. He is young and hip. The kind of guy you would not be surprised to find working in, well, a cool Parisian bookstore.

"It is amazing how many current bands have adopted this sound," I say in an effort to stimulate further discussion. The checkout guy seems friendly and genuinely interested, so I continue. "Like, for example, the band Beach House. Much of their stuff has a big *Pet Sounds* vibe."

"Funny you should say that," the hip book salesman replies. "I was the drummer for Beach House."

To truly appreciate the otherworldly weirdness of this coincidence, consider the following facts. Both Adam and I love Beach House. It is a band that has ascended to the very pinnacle of the critical-acclaim heap. For those of you who do not follow the current music scene, imagine that this were the 1970s, and you discovered a member of The Ramones, Talking Heads or The Velvet Underground working as a clerk in a bookstore. I am not saying that Beach House is going to have that kind of staying power and long-term cultural influence, but this gives you a sense of where the band currently sits in the musical hierarchy. All of their albums have ended up on "best of" lists. Many critics picked their album, *Bloom*, as the best album of 2012. And one well-known list that uses a complex formula to correlate reviews and rankings has them as a respectable 160th best band of *all time*. This is just fourteen places below Madonna, five below Public Enemy and three below Cream.

From the outside looking in, Beach House seems like a commercially successful outfit. They've played on David Letterman and regularly sell out medium-sized venues all over the world. When I think of a "Beach House lifestyle," I think tour buses, personal assistants and nice hotels. A rock 'n' roll existence. So you won't be surprised to know that my first thought is, *Yeah right, I'm sure you were the drummer for Beach House*. And that my second thought, which comes after some further banter that had the not-so-well-hidden goal of confirming the veracity of the drummer's claim, is, *What the hell is a bona fide rock star doing working in a bookstore?*

DREAMS OF FAME AND FORTUNE

Twenty-five years ago the top-five career ambitions of grade school children were teacher, banker, doctor, scientist and vet. Now, according to a recent survey from the UK, they are, in descending order of awesomeness, sports star, pop star, actor, astronaut and lawyer. While "lawyer" may seem reasonably sensible (hey, *I'm* a lawyer!), I suspect most of these kids have no interest in being a real lawyer. They aren't dreaming of working ninety hours a week on personal injury cases for a soul-sucking law firm. They don't want to drag their butts out of bed at 5:30 A.M. to get in a few extra billable hours. They don't want to babysit two hundred or so mind-numbingly boring client files. They want to be the slick, fast-talking, well-dressed and sexy TV-drama version of a lawyer. (I can personally confirm that this version does not exist in the real world.)

The dream of celebrity and fame endures well into late adolescence. Another UK study, involving more than one thousand sixteen-year-olds, found that more than half had fame as their primary career goal. Other UK research, in 2006, has found that 16 percent of sixteen- to nineteen-year-olds believed they were going to be famous. Eleven percent were ready to quit school to pursue this goal. My daughter, Alison, was sufficiently surprised by these numbers that she queried her twenty-six grade nine classmates about their aspirations. More than 50 percent of them told her that they were hoping for a celebrity-oriented profession. Six saw themselves becoming actors; five, professional athletes; and several, film directors. Only one in this class of relatively affluent children wanted to be a scientist, which is a bit ironic, given that the school sits blocks from my university's huge new biomedical research building. One student is hoping to be a doctor and another is aiming for teaching—drama, naturally. One said he wanted to be an explosives expert. (Is that a job?)

Jake Halpern surveyed 650 US teenagers for his book *Fame Junkies*. A remarkable 43.4 percent aspired to be an assistant to a "very famous singer or movie star." By comparison, 23.7 percent said they wanted to be "the president of a great university like Harvard or Yale"; 13.6 percent saw themselves as "a United States Senator"; 9.8 percent as a "Navy SEAL"; and 9.5 percent as head of a major company. Think about that. Four out of ten teenagers would rather get coffee, make appointments and pick up dry cleaning for a celebrity than have their own prestigious and rewarding career!

The bottom line: fame and celebrity status are now *the* dominant ambitions. Kids just want to be famous. And a growing body of research supports this finding. A 2011 study, for example, found that fame was the number-one cultural value of children between the ages of ten and twelve. The kids in this study were asked to think about their future and the traits they would like to possess: the desire to be famous was their top choice. Indeed, the abstract notion of fame—the desire simply to be known by a large number of strangers—as a future goal ranked well above being kind, successful, having love and acceptance or, even, being rich. And, perhaps most interesting, the researcher found that none of the children in the study, not a single one, mentioned a particular skill or talent associated with the concept of fame. Not one said he or she wanted to excel at a sport or at acting. Another study asked ten-year-olds what they believed would be "the very best thing

in the world." The number one answer: "Being a celebrity."
"Friends" ranked seventh.

One of the most comprehensive research projects on point
was conducted in Tasmania, Australia, in 2011. The researchers
asked more than one thousand primary school children about
their hopes and dreams. Once again, fame and celebrity were
the overriding themes. A few youngsters were aiming for prime
minister, but, in general, the kids wanted to be entertainment
and sports stars. For part of the study they were asked to draw
a picture of a leaf with their hopes for the future written inside.
Some were general. Versions of the nebulous "I want to be
famous" were common. Others were pretty specific. One grade
six boy, for example, said he wanted "to be an actor and to
live in Los Angeles and to have a lovely wife and two children
living the high life." (That does sound like a mighty fine
lifestyle.) Many of the kids saw music as their portal to fame.
Here are two of my favorite quotes, both from grade six boys:
"My hope is that my band makes it into the big bucks and
famous. Rock on!" and "I would like to be rich with a big
mansion. To become a well-known musician that plays in a
band." I love these statements because they could have been
made by the grade six me and also, as it turns out, by many, if
not most, of the musicians I spoke with while researching this
book, including, I bet, the Parisian bookstore clerk and former
Beach House drummer.

In this part of the book, I seek to shed some light on the reality
of the fame game and the drive for celebrity. We will see that

everything is an illusion. Not only is no pot of gold waiting at the end of the rainbow (well, very rarely, a pot does await, but it usually isn't filled with the promised, happiness-inducing gold) but also the rainbow isn't real. It is a projection created by the market, the media and our own cognitive and biologically determined predisposition, and our hopes and dreams. Moreover, I will argue, believing in the existence of the celebrity rainbow has numerous adverse consequences.

It may seem, at least initially, that this section is a real downer. Pulling the curtain back on the illusion of celebrity can come off a bit frosty. My younger brother, Sean, was sent home from kindergarten once for running a recess seminar on his "There is no Santa Claus" theory, which was largely based on the hypothesis that Christmas is a capitalist plot designed to sell lots of toys. (I wonder who forced these radical ideas into his impressionable five-year-old brain?) I don't want to be *that* guy now. I don't want to kill Santa Claus. Big dreams, even if unrealistic, are fun and can play an important social role. Plus, I can completely relate to the fantasy of fame. I devoted a significant part of my young adult life to the pursuit of rock 'n' roll stardom.

But more importantly, I believe the message of this section is liberating. Ideally, it will release us from the grip of celebrity-fueled ambitions and the social expectations that come with them. I hope it allows us to make more informed choices as individuals and parents. More broadly, I hope it highlights the pernicious impact of celebrity culture on our values and our conception of the good life.

One can become a celebrity in a whole bunch of ways. There are famous authors (though not many, and the benefits conferred on them by fame usually are modest). There are famous politicians (though that doesn't seem like a fun kind of fame). And there are even famous scientists (again, not many). In this era, however, I think most people associate fame and celebrity with several fairly specific activities: music, acting, sports and, um, nothing (the relatively new famous-for-being-famous gig). These are the avenues to fame most often mentioned by children and adolescents. Rock star! Movie star! Sports star! So, these are the areas I focus on in my attempt to show how illusory they really are.

Of course, young people are not the only ones yearning for celebrity status. Other research tells us that fame remains the number-one goal for a significant number of adults; hence the steady stream of reality show applicants. A recent survey from the US found that fame and celebrity increasingly have become what people view as the "American Dream." It is never too late to be famous, I guess. As I mentioned, I held on to my rock star dreams well into my twenties. In fact, I think my twenty-sixth birthday was my most depressing, far more so than when I turned thirty or forty. Those later birthdays breezed by without a drop of age-related despondency. But my twenty-sixth was the year that I had a full-on existential crisis. It was the year I realized I would never be the front man of a monstrously successful and critically acclaimed rock band. That dream, alas, was dead.

It's not just kids whose imaginations are fired up by the prospect of fame. Many parents see some form of celebrity—athlete, actor or pop star—as the most desirable career option for their children. For some, seeking celebrity has become a central family activity, one that consumes a significant amount of their financial resources and their time. Is all this striving, whether for yourself or your children, folly? Can we all really become celebrities if we just keep dreaming big and reaching for the stars?

CHAPTER 7

SO YOU WANT TO BE A STAR?

ROCK STAR!

My flight to the Austin, Texas, South by Southwest (SXSW) music festival was non-stop from New York's JFK. Judging by the number of guitar cases, the quantity of DJ gear, the predominance of I-wish-I-didn't-have-to-get-up expressions on people's faces and the answers to a few random queries, the boarding area was overflowing with musicians. The crowd included a smattering of fans, business executives, music lawyers and people involved in music promotion, but mostly it was bedraggled individuals wearing attire that unimaginatively advertised their musical affiliation: hip hop, alt country, rock 'n' roll, retro punk, ironic quirky pop, etc. The plane at the gate next to our flight was heading to Florida and the slow-moving passenger line was peppered with wheelchairs, Bermuda shorts and polo shirts. The contrast with the hipster caravan I was about to join could not have been starker. One line filled with retirees, the other with people who probably rarely think about that kind of late-life lifestyle.

SXSW is billed as the world's largest music conference or, as their website declares, the "biggest and most anticipated convergence of all things music." More than two thousand "official" musical acts show up to play at hundreds of venues—large, medium and rumpus-room-ish in dimension—throughout the downtown core. The roster includes well-established big-name bands, up-and-coming acts and bands that are new but have lots of buzz. (I heard the word "buzz" hundreds of times while at SXSW, as in: "no buzz," "buzz-less," "about to catch some buzz," "no point in coming unless you have buzz" and the much coveted "buzz band.") Hundreds, perhaps thousands, of unofficial acts also play in unofficial (rough, closet-size) venues.

While the music is the focus and the public draw, the music industry people I spoke with told me that SXSW is really a big schmooze-fest industry party. Given this fine mandate, it seemed an ideal place to explore the state of the music industry and its role in the celebrity game. Specifically, I wanted to explore the current status of the celebrity musician. Is the rock star job still available? And, more broadly, can you get rich and famous in music?

My guide for the event is a good friend, CJ Murdoch—aka Cecil Frena, Edmonton's electro-pop music wiz and leader of the one-man-band Born Gold. CJ's career path might be considered eccentric by some. He was a rising star in the world of legal academia. He obtained a law degree from the University of Alberta, worked at a U of A research centre, published a number of well-received academic articles, was given a fellowship at Stanford University and, just a few years ago, gave it all up. CJ went all in. He doesn't do music as a hobby or as a part-time job. He is a full-time, struggling musician. And wow! The vast majority of professional musicians do *struggle*.

In March 2013 the Canadian Independent Music Association released a comprehensive report on the economic impact of the music industry. The message was pretty clear. If getting rich and famous is your goal, pick a different profession. The average income for an independent musician in Canada is $7228 per year. Yes, per *year*. That is less than half of the Canadian poverty line cutoff, and about $4000 less than the average US poverty cutoff (which varies from state to state). And we aren't talking about garage bands whose members are attending the local community college and living at home with mom and dad. The average age of these impoverished minstrels was thirty-nine (I suppose they could still be at home with mom and dad) and the average-size audience they played to was well over seven hundred. These are people putting in full-time or near full-time hours. These are real, touring, hardworking, professional musicians. The kind you pay good money to see. The kind who play at SXSW, have cool T-shirts (an important source of income!), and who you hear on public radio.

"Um, that number seems about right," CJ told me over the thump of an electro-pop band from Montreal. We were standing with a group of musicians at a SXSW venue dedicated to music from Quebec. "Actually, after a rough calculation of my own expenses and income, I'd say I am just about average! Hilarious." Bear in mind that CJ has achieved what seems like a reasonable amount of success. He has headlined festivals, toured the world, had his songs licensed for TV spots and received a good deal of positive coverage from the international music press.

As I went from venue to venue—using CJ as my backstage pass—I ran these numbers by various musicians, both experienced and inexperienced, from all over North America and got the same that's-about-right reaction. Some were initially shocked, many laughed at the absurdity of their situation, but after a bit of reflection, everyone agreed that the depressing numbers provided by the Canadian Independent Music Association rang true. You might be thinking, sure, independent musicians don't make much. They are, after all, *independent* musicians. In order to catch the celebrity-propelling brass ring, you need to sign a record deal with a big label. Well, you're both right and wrong.

It's true that the chance of making it really big without industry money is remote. One analysis of the UK music scene concluded that your chance of financial "success" (modestly defined as making the national average income for *one year*!) without a major record deal is next to zero. After considering the number of "serious" musicians in the UK and the money generated from paying gigs and downloads, the author concluded that the chance of making an average income for just one year was a stupefyingly unlikely 0.0025 percent. But even if you snag an industry record deal, you have absolutely no guarantee you will make any money or get close to achieving celebrity.

Moses Avalon, a well-known music industry expert and commentator, has written several books on the music scene, including the often-referenced *Confessions of a Record Producer: How to Survive the Scams and Shams of the Music Business.* He is a fearless skeptic and crusader for artists' rights, and so he seemed to be an ideal person to approach about the reality of rock 'n' roll stardom. More importantly, not long ago he did an impressive analysis of the very issue I was exploring: the chances of making it big with a major label deal.

Moses estimates that out of the 43,000 submissions that go to major labels each year, only 1 in 2149 will make it through a multiple-album deal, which is probably what is required to achieve what he calls a "quitting-your-day-job" standard of living. In other words, only .047 percent will have anything close to a stable career. (Many commentators think that Moses' already bleak number is, in fact, *too* optimistic, because they figure the number of submissions, if you include all the basement tape demos, is much greater.) While these odds are terrifyingly slim, Moses notes that they are better than trying to stay indie. According to his analysis, based on the "raw odds," as Moses says, of selling about five thousand units for several albums in a row, what are the chances of quitting-your-day-job indie success? 1 in 477,000! As Moses notes, it may not be one in a million, but from the perspective of a struggling indie artist, it might as well be. When I called to ask about his analysis, he immediately displayed his pull-no-punches approach to life. He said he didn't like my first question about the chance of making it celebrity big. "I don't want to tell you how to do an interview.... But what the hell do you mean by 'celebrity rock star'? Every singer in a band thinks he is a rock star."

Good point.

"Look, it has *always* been near impossible to become a true, Jagger-style rock star," Moses continued. "That is a billion-to-one phenomenon. It just doesn't happen. Let's talk about just making a living. Many musicians don't realize how tough it is to make a reasonable income in this industry."

I told Moses that many of the industry people I chatted with at SXSW thought that the age of the celebrity rock star might be over—at least for the foreseeable future. But they also talked about the rise of the middle-class band, suggesting that while there are few big stars, more are making a solid, middle-class income. "How the hell do they define 'middle class'?" Moses replied. "Could you raise a family on the money they are talking about? No."

Again, good point.

In fact, there is scant evidence of a growing middle-class or, even, lower-middle-class bulge of musicians. On the contrary, just as in the broader economy, fewer musicians seem to be taking a big hunk of the available revenue. A 2013 analysis of the music industry, this one by Princeton economist and chair of the Council of Economic Advisers Alan B. Krueger, identified a winner-take-all trend in the music industry, one that parallels what is happening in most countries' economies. Few are truly rich and those few are getting richer. For example, as Krueger notes, "The share of concert revenue taken home by the top 1 percent of performers has more than doubled, rising from 26 percent in 1982 to 56 percent in 2003 … [and] the top 5 percent take home almost 90 percent of all concert revenues."

On my flight to Austin I sat between a record company executive and a well-known lawyer from New York who represents musicians (both asked to remain anonymous). For much of the flight they good-naturedly entertained my naive questions about the industry. At one point they produced a long list of bands performing at SXSW. It was their must-see list. I asked the lawyer to name a band that was making a comfortable income—one that had passed the quit-your-day-job threshold. She ran her finger down the list. "Nope, nope, nope," she said. And then, with raised eyebrows, "None." Remember, these are hot bands—buzz bands—invited to play at one of the world's biggest music events.

While it has always been difficult to make money in the music business, there are many reasons why the path to success is likely bumpier now than ever before. One is the profound fragmentation of the market. When I was in high school—admittedly, a long time ago—the genres were, basically, pop, rock, country, folk, funk and soul. There was a radio station for each and record stores (remember them?) that divided their stock into these broad categories. Now it seems as if there are countless genres and sub-genres. A Wikipedia page on music genres lists more than 170—for electronic music alone! While this fragmentation is great for consumers looking for a sound that fits a very specific taste (for example, chill wave, darkcore, happy hardcore, ghettotech, space disco or futurepop), it has resulted in a vast number of small markets, which, arguably, makes the sale of tons of product to a broad audience tough.

There is also a crazy amount of product out there. The competition for ear time is stiff. About seventy-five thousand albums are released each year (up from around thirty thousand a decade ago). Few of those sell. At all. In 2009, for example, only 2.1 percent of all the albums released that year sold more than five thousand copies. While that is bleak, a closer look at the numbers paints an even gloomier picture. Ninety-four percent of new releases (album or single) sold fewer than a thousand copies and 80 percent sold fewer than a hundred. *Fewer than a hundred!* If you discount the copies sold to family and friends, then most artists are selling zilch. Zero. And, keep in mind, even if you do sell a reasonable number and are lucky enough to have a major label deal, the notoriously crappy contract you signed means that you will make almost nothing. There are many mouths to feed in the music business and everyone has found a way to take a bite out of the revenue pie. One calculation suggests that after taking out the money that goes to the label, the lawyers, the distributors, etc., the average musician nets just $23 for every $1000 of gross receipts. As I said, depressing.

"If you are really, really lucky, you can live comfortably for a while—maybe making fifty thousand [a year] for a few years—but it can't be sustained. Almost no one continues to make that kind of money," Greg Paquet told me. Greg has been in the music business for more than a decade. He was the guitar player in the successful Canadian band The Stills. Now, by "successful" I mean that he seemed successful by the outside-looking-in criteria. The band, which broke up in 2011, toured the world, played to huge audiences (in 2010, for example, they toured with the arena rock band Kings of Leon), had singles that got frequent radio play (such as their catchy 2003 tune, "Still in Love Song"), garnered great reviews and awards (in 2009, The Stills won a Juno for best Canadian alternative band), opened for Paul McCartney (!) and, if you believe Greg, made very little money. "The reality stinks. When you hit your late twenties, you must make a choice," the past-his-late-twenties Greg told me. He is currently playing bass for the Quebec singer Peter Peter. I saw him play at a late-afternoon showcase at SXSW. There were about thirty people in the room. But those thirty were enthusiastic and the band was seriously terrific. Greg seemed to be having a good time. I guess he has made his—rather well-informed—choice.

For many of the SXSW artists I chatted with, merely surviving has become the primary goal. The dream of fame and fortune often burns bright, but reality is never far from view. Another artist, the respected electronic musician who performs under the name Baths, put it this way: "When I was a kid, I wanted to be a rock star, then I wanted to be a successful musician, and then I just wanted paying work. You downsize your expectations. Not artistically, but in terms of fame and money. Now I just want to be a bit comfortable. I want to get to a place where everything in my life isn't falling apart."

Of course, the paths to fame and fortune in the music industry are many and varied. Thanks to shows such as *American Idol*, the way can seem tremendously short and spectacularly direct. The premise of the show, and of all its imitators, is that contestants have the chance to realize their dreams instantly. But what is the likelihood that a show such as *Idol* will propel a person to celebrity status? Pretty darn small.

My eldest son, Adam, analyzed the careers of the *Idol* contestants who finished in the top twelve in the first five seasons. I asked Adam to do this for two reasons. First, he's cheap labor. Second, I wanted to access his teenage sensibilities in the assessment of whether a contestant was successful. I wanted to know if, through the eyes of a media-saturated teenager, a given *Idol* contestant was celebrity big. For each contestant, Adam looked through Twitter, iTunes and other relevant websites (e.g., the Internet Movie Database). He looked for stories about their careers, record contracts, involvement in Broadway productions, etc. We then worked together to give each Idol a ranking, from a Carrie Underwood high (as the most successful Idol ever, she gets a rank of 10) to singing-on-a-cruise-ship low. What did we find? While many *Idol* finalists are working in the entertainment industry, *very* few have found anything close to what could be considered big-time success. Out of the fifty-eight finalists tracked (the first season had ten), Kelly Clarkson, Clay Aiken, Ruben Studdard, Jennifer Hudson, Fantasia Barrino, Carrie Underwood, Chris Daughtry, Katharine McPhee and Taylor Hicks rated as an 8 or above. These are the few that have relatively broad name recognition and reasonably solid careers. Others, such as Mandisa from season 5 (Christian music) and Constantine Maroulis from season 4 (musical theater), are doing well, but I think this is a fair list of the contestants who can be classed as truly successful by industry standards. (One could argue that we were overly generous in our assessment of Hicks, Studdard and Barrino—none of my kids had ever heard of them. Ditto my kids' friends.)

It is difficult to find the exact number of people who try out for *Idol*, but estimates range from 50,000 to 100,000 per season. So altogether, approximately 200,000 to 300,000 people likely auditioned in those first five years. This means those who audition have about a 9 in 250,000 chance of achieving celebrity success through *Idol*. Once again, this means, from the perspective of a practical assessment of your odds, that your chance might as well be zero. Even if we take a very conservative approach and guesstimate that only 1 out of every 100 who audition sing well enough to be in the mix, and suppose for the sake of argument that you are one of them, this still translates into about a 0.36 percent chance of a career that will fall somewhere between Taylor Hicks's and Carrie Underwood's. In other words, even the top 1 percent of *Idol* contestants have a slim chance of celebrity success.

Of course, we need to be careful in our definition of "success"—a point I will return to below. Here, I am talking about making it celebrity big, not some form of artistic success—which is, of course, a critical distinction, particularly in the world of reality TV.

I interviewed Lisa Leuschner, an *Idol* semifinalist from season 3. The woman can sing. Indeed, she has been called "the most prematurely, unjustly eliminated contestant in show history"; her performance of "Sweet Thing" was an *Idol* standout. But despite her obvious talent and comfort on the stage, the judges voted her off the show. (It is worth noting that on an earlier show one of the judges—Simon Cowell, no surprise—commented on her weight, suggesting she was too big to be an *Idol*. It is unclear whether this is the reason she was voted off.) Despite this, she isn't bitter about her *Idol* ride, mostly because she seems to have a remarkably clearheaded appreciation—at least for someone who has invested time in *American Idol*—of the nature of the music industry. This is due, no doubt, to her extensive pre-*Idol* experience as a working singer. I asked her why so many people continue to audition for the show. "Many of the kids on *Idol* [are] caught up in the star thing," Leuschner tells me. "Many have no idea what it is like to be a musician. It is not an easy job. It is hard work. But I have no regrets. I feel blessed to be a working singer. That's who I am."

Leuschner continues to be employed—performing mostly blues and gospel. As of this writing (and I am streaming her amazing voice as I type these words) she is touring with the band Foreverland, a tribute to Michael Jackson. Leuschner's experience highlights a point that should be abundantly clear by now: raw ability and hard work are absolutely no guarantee of success on *Idol* or in the music industry generally. If you define success as doing something you love, Leuschner is doing just fine. The problem is that in the world of celebrity wannabes, success is rarely defined in such sensible terms. Anything other than stardom can be cast as a failure.

I ask another former *Idol*, Martin Kerr, about our culture's fame-focused standard of success. Kerr finished in the top sixteen of the now defunct Canadian version of the show and has since carved out a solid singing career. While far from famous, Kerr tells me he has attained what most would consider a middle-class lifestyle. And he has achieved this, not by selling CDs or touring the world, but by playing "local farmers' markets, churches, schools, house concerts, weddings, festivals, charity and corporate events, stuff that many musicians don't even consider doing." He is entirely satisfied with his music career and is frustrated because most people view success in terms of fame and fortune. "I think it's strange that we judge success in music by a different yardstick than other industries," Kerr notes. "If you work in IT and make a good living at it, people consider you a success. They don't say, 'keep trying' or 'I hope you make it someday' because you're not Bill Gates. But if you do the same in music, people say exactly those things until they've seen you on MTV."

MOVIE STAR!

The best estimates I could find suggest that about thirty thousand professional actors live in New York City. At the same time, according to some calculations, about eight hundred good jobs are available for them, ranging from off-Broadway bit parts to steady chorus line work to leads in major productions. Not a lot of jobs for an awful lot of actors. And the thirty thousand number includes only those actors who hold membership in one of the relevant unions—individuals who are, generally, experienced and, arguably, employable. If you include all the other actors struggling to get a paying gig who are not yet part of a union—assuming the three-to-one ratio suggested to me by several actors—then we are closing in on a final count of around a hundred thousand desperate thespians. I met one of them in a bar overlooking Union Square.

Ramesh Ganeshram is a good-looking guy. He clearly satisfies the actor-must-be-at-least-kinda-hot criterion. Also, he has a hard-to-pin-down ethnicity. Is he Indian? Arab? Ethiopian? (As he later joked, "I can play everything from evil terrorist to non-threatening friendly ethnic neighbor to everything in between—it is a good time for a guy like me!") These luck-of-the-draw genetic characteristics must, I suppose (somewhat uncomfortably), help to set him apart from at least a few of the hundred thousand.

Ramesh gives me a warm hello and firm handshake. He seems to be an ideal case study for this book. He is your typical working actor, still struggling to "make it big." We settle into our booth and he starts telling me about his career, the various acting schools and classes he has attended, the theater work in which he has performed, the bit parts he has played in independent movies, and so on, but he seems more than a little distracted. It turns out that he had an audition earlier that day for the popular NBC TV show *Law and Order SVU*. It was a small part, but a good one. It was network TV, paid real money and would be a great addition to his résumé. He wanted it. Badly. It was going to be tough for him to relax, he informs me after a long soul-centering sigh, until he hears how the audition went. This is understandable. I order a beer. He orders green tea.

Acting, like singing and playing in a band, is, in reality, an unbelievable, spirit-crushing grind. It might be even worse than the music business. Music you can do on your own. You can play on the street. You can use social media to build an audience. But with acting—unless we are talking about the "acting" that takes place sans clothes for a paying internet audience—you need other people. You need a stage or a camera or, at least, a classroom filled with like-minded colleagues willing to indulge your need to perform. I think almost everyone knows this. It is a fairly accepted reality that acting is a tough way to put food on the table. A million or so jokes poke fun at how chronically unemployed actors are. (An actor says to his friends at a restaurant: "Good news! I got another callback. My agent says it's between me and the guy who's going to get it!") Still, given that one of the goals of this chapter is to inject a bit of cold realism into the subject, and given that tens of thousands of individuals hope to use acting as a path—either for themselves or their talented offspring—to celebrity status, it is worth some further exploration.

While we sip our drinks, Ramesh tells me about the many things he must do to keep his acting career moving: acting lessons, off-off-off-Broadway productions, constant hustling and, naturally, innumerable auditions. One night he performed in front of *one* person—and she was the girlfriend of a cast member. But this is what he loves. At this point, he can't do acting full-time, which is the norm for most of the people who describe themselves as actors, so he does have a day job. But he is quick to point out that the day job is only to pay the rent. It's not a plan B. "You can't have a plan B; otherwise you are going to fail," he explains. He's "all in."

I heard this "No Plan B" theory from another, very successful (i.e., lead in movies and TV shows) actor. The idea is that having a plan B both compromises your craft and undermines your chance of success. It is as if the "Success Gods" are watching and will reward only those who are fully committed. No one deserves entry into the realm of stardom unless they have truly suffered. "I constantly wonder what else I should be doing. Should I move to LA? Some actors tell me I must move because that is the logical next step. That is where the jobs are. Others say I should stay in New York because there is too much competition in LA." Ramesh isn't kidding: there is a lot of competition in LA. It has been estimated that LA is home to about three times the number of actors living in New York. Ramesh is just starting to catch his stride in what I sense is a well-rehearsed rant about the challenges of being an actor in New York when he freezes mid-sentence.

"Damn! Damn! Where is it?" He suddenly becomes aware that his cell phone is not within earshot. He frantically does the universally familiar cell-phone-search dance. The entire routine is completed within seconds. Front pants pockets. Nope. Back pants pockets. Nope. Shirt pocket. Nope. Jacket. Bingo! And then he stares wide-eyed at the phone. He missed a call. He missed *the* call. "I can't believe it! I've carried this fucking phone with me all day. I even stared at it while I was in the bathroom. I am so sorry. I gotta call them back right now!" He pops out of our booth and executes a quick zigzag exit from the bar, cell phone at his ear.

What are the chances Ramesh will become a "star," which, he had no hesitation admitting, he would "absolutely love and any actor who says otherwise is a liar"? If we define "star" as a highly paid studio-movie actor, his chances are ridiculously, infinitesimally tiny. While I couldn't find any hardcore academic research on point, several examinations of the issue have been released in the popular press. For example, the *Book of Odds* uses the Ulmer Scale (a well-known industry list of Hollywood's hottest actors) to put the chances at an incomprehensibly unlikely 1 in 1,505,000. You have a much better chance of getting killed by an asteroid (about 1 in 700,000). Other, more forgiving calculations take into account that if you are a serious, full-time actor, you really aren't competing against everyone dreaming of being a Hollywood star, just other serious, full-time actors. Still, every calculation I found framed the chances as so remote that if we were talking about an adverse event (such as being struck by lightning) instead of a reaching-for-the-stars ambition (becoming a well-paid actor), we would simply say *not going to happen*. True, these kinds of rough calculations are hardly scientifically robust, particularly since, as noted, the denominator includes more than just seriously committed actors. And, of course, a huge amount of luck, timing and genetics (do you look like a movie star?) is involved—a point I will return to below—that can raise or lower your chances. Just the same, these figures help to convey the rarity of making it celebrity big in the acting game.

The statistics related to child actors are slightly more concrete, mostly because the field is somewhat regulated and, as a result, more statistics are available, but they're equally gloomy. Each year there are, for example, more than twenty thousand child actors, just counting those with agents, in the Hollywood area alone. If you include *all* the child actors looking for work, the number is likely much larger. I saw one calculation, based on child work permits, that put the number at more than sixty thousand. This city-sized horde of aspiring and parent-ally "encouraged" celebrity wannabes is scrambling for about twenty-five regular TV roles. And a lot of people in the industry, including a former child star, told me that almost all those parts go to kids who already have a significant acting résumé. If your child does not already have solid showbiz credits to his or her name, his or her chance of getting a job is, as succinctly summar-ized by BizParent, a foundation dedicated to supporting children in the entertainment industry, "almost zip."

"Sorry about the frantic arrival. I was just at an audition for some God-awful big budget *roooobot* movie. Even after thirty years, nothing changes. You must audition!"

What's up with actors? It seems that every one I meet is *just* coming from an audition. This robot-movie auditioner is the versatile thespian Michael Simkins. We meet in a charming hotel bar close to Victoria Station in London. Michael isn't breaking any respected-middle-aged British actor stereotypes. And I mean that in the nicest way possible. He is fun, witty and articulate. The kind of guy you'd like to have a few pints with. I am thrilled to have the opportunity to chat with Michael. In acting terms, he has done it all. He has been in successful West End theater productions, such as *Chicago* and *Mamma Mia!* He has been in big-budget movies, such as *The Iron Lady* and *V Is for Vendetta*. He has been a semi-regular on a TV show, including a recent stint on the popular UK show *EastEnders*. And he has been through the early-career acting grind, which included performing in more than sixty plays in five years. (He can still, from memory, list them all.) While not quite a celebrity, he is, by almost any measure, a successful working actor. Or, as he puts it, "I am a man who has spent his life somewhere between triumph and complete oblivion." More importantly for me, he has put a great deal of thought into the challenges of being an actor. He has written two books and numerous editorials, mostly for *The Guardian*, on his craft. Indeed, for the UK media, he is one of the go-to commentators for all things acting—a status that is confirmed during our discussion by a call from a reporter for meaty actor-ish quotes on some urgent theatrical development.

"Impossible goal. Simply impossible."

This is Michael's quick response when I ask him if my new friend Ramesh had a chance of becoming a movie star. I run the better-chance-of-getting-hit-by-an-asteroid factoid by him. "That sounds about right," he says after a pause. "The problem, of course, is that it *does* happen. There are some new actors that make it. Proof that it happens is on TV and in movies. We *see* them succeed. We are dazzled by the possibilities. This allows us to hold on to the dream that we could be the next one. This makes it hard to be realistic."

Okay, if we are being realistic, Ramesh has, basically, no measurable chance of becoming a celebrity actor. But what are his chances of becoming a well-paid, comfortable working actor, such as the genial man sitting across from me in the London bar? While the point here is that using acting as a vehicle to celebrity is folly, it is worth noting that even this far more modest goal is hard. It has been said—not coincidentally, by Michael Simkins in an editorial he wrote for *The Guardian*—that actor employment statistics are terrifying, "with something like 92% of the profession out of work at any one time." To make matters worse, the same 8 percent tend to get much of the work. So the key is to break into the 8 percent and stay there, always bearing in mind that the vast majority of this 8 percent don't make much money.

But life as one of the 8 percent is only rarely celebrity posh. As one New York–based actress who asked to remain anonymous (a common request by actors who comment on their profession) told me, "Your job as an actor is, basically, rejection and auditioning … and more rejection. There is very little actual acting." This is a woman who is in the we-should-hire-her loop and, as such, she gets fairly regular jobs and just a few weeks before our discussion auditioned for, but did not get, a substantial role in a Hollywood blockbuster. Michael agrees with her assessment. In fact, he goes further. "If I had to provide a definition of a professional actor, I'd say it is someone who is prepared to live with *no*, and to live with *daily* rejection," he says with a dramatic emphasis.

To make this story even more depressing for all the aspiring actors out there, the quick churn created by our modern celebrity culture and the growing legions of celebrity-seeking actors is making it even more difficult to get established. "To be honest, if you are a new actor," Michael tells me, "your best chance of making it [as a working actor] is in the first fourteen to sixteen months you are on the scene. You are fresh. Agents and casting directors are looking for something new and exciting. If you haven't gotten established in this brief time span, you've got to compete with the next vomit of actors pouring out of acting schools everywhere around the world. You aren't new anymore."

❖

Back in New York I watch Ramesh pace back and forth on the sidewalk just outside the bar talking on his phone. His body language provides no clue about how the audition went. There is no fist pumping or Rocky pose. My guess: no job. Woody Allen famously wrote, "Show business is not so much dog eats dog, as dog doesn't return other dog's phone calls." I figure that it is terrific that, at least, Ramesh got a chance to audition and no matter what news was being conveyed, he has taken another step in the right direction. At least the dog returned his call. I start thinking about the best way to say "too bad" without sounding like a condescending dick.

Ramesh steps back into the bar. One look at his face and I know my guess was wrong. He got the part. From a selfish point of view, I can't believe my luck. To actually *witness* an actor get a job is a bit like seeing a meteorite hit the ground. You know it happens—the Earth is covered in craters—but to be there when a call arrives seems too good to be true.

"Wow, we shoot on Monday," Ramesh says with a wide smile. He pushes his green tea aside and orders a beer. "This is a great profession." Time to celebrate. The dream lives on.

SPORTS STAR!

Of course, music and acting are just two of the ways people think about getting famous. Another perceived path to celebrity is through achievement in sports. Indeed, for many young athletes, "going pro" is viewed as an entirely sensible ambition. And, sadly, many parents hold this view as well. In reality, the chance of making it as a sports celebrity, like the chance of making it as an actor, is almost zip. For example, a kid in Canada playing in minor league hockey right now has a much better chance of getting struck by lightning or dying of flesh-eating disease than of playing a single game in the NHL—even if the kid has been identified as talented, is currently a minor league star and has all the right support and training. An often-quoted 1999 analysis looked, retrospectively, at a group of 30,000 kids playing minor hockey in Southern Ontario. Of that number, 235 were drafted into the Ontario Hockey League (the minor league), but only 110 of those got to play and even fewer, 90, played for more than three years. Of course, the number for those who made it to the NHL—a step necessary in order to have a sports career that would confer "celebrity" status—was even smaller. Fifty of the 30,000 were drafted, but only 25 played a game. (As it happens, even this number was unusually high—it was a good year.) If you look at the number of players who had something close to what could be called a "career"—which, in this study, meant players still in the league at age twenty-four—the number drops to just 11. Bottom line: only 11 out of 30,000 ended up with a solid NHL career. And that was in 1999. Because more professional players are now coming from countries other than Canada, it is even more difficult to break in.

If you want to look at this from a cold statistical stand-point, you *cannot* become rich and famous from professional sports. It is so rare, as is the case with becoming a movie or rock star, it borders on the statistically impossible. Technically, something is only statistically impossible if the chances of it happening are zero, but 11 out of 30,000 is getting darn close to zero. It is .037 percent. And comparably grim numbers exist for other sports, such as basketball and football. If you take the high school seniors playing on school teams as the denominator, and generally these are fairly serious athletes, there is only a .03 percent chance of a pro career in basketball. Out of 156,000 high school senior basketball players, only 44 will be drafted to play in the NBA after college. Similarly, there is a .08 percent chance of a pro career in football. Out of 317,000 high school senior football players, approximately 250 get drafted. And it should not be forgotten that "getting drafted" is no guarantee of a career. On the contrary, obscurity is the norm for most draftees.

CHAPTER 8

CELEBRITY DREAMS AND COGNITIVE BIASES

Not everyone is pursuing celebrity. When measured against the entire population, the number of individuals who are committed to becoming an actor, singer or sports star is not huge. One commentator estimated that, in 2009, approximately four million adults in the United States had fame as their primary and explicit goal. Add children and adolescents and that number increases substantially. And, I am guessing, the number likely doesn't include those seeking sports fame, because the goal of becoming a professional athlete is often not characterized as a celebrity ambition. In addition, as noted by the well-known human development scholar Oliver Gilbert Brim, "there is an unknown but substantial number of people with the fame motive who deny it to the world and keep it a secret even to themselves." In other words, the pursuit of celebrity may be an unconscious or covert motivator for many people. We may not want to admit it, but the idea of celebrity and fame may, nevertheless, shape how we think about our goals, activities and current lot in life.

The belief that fame and celebrity are sensible life options has broad social ramifications. And, while the number of individuals actually committed to chasing fame is comparatively small, it is also not insignificant. Even if you accept the conservative calculation put forward by Brim, that there are four million fame seekers in America alone, this is still a phenomenal number of individuals who will not achieve the celebrity status they so desperately desire, and who are spending their valuable time on this Earth in an utterly futile pursuit.

Indeed, Brim provides yet another example of the massive disconnect between the desire for fame and the actual chance of achieving it. (I promise, this is my last bit of you-ain't-gonna-make-it statistical dream crushing.) Drawing on a number of sources, including the number of hall of fame biographical entries for the fame-related professions, Brim estimated that about twenty thousand "fame slots" are open to the four million fame seekers. (I think this is an overly generous calculation, as not all hall of fame actors, singers or, even, athletes are true celebrities, but supposing he's right, 3,980,000 remain who are going to be seriously disappointed.) So, we know the chances of grabbing the brass ring are slim, and we know that eager hordes keep reaching for it. It is, then, worth considering the cognitive and social forces that keep the celebrity dream alive. Why do so many people believe, despite all the evidence to the contrary, that they're going to be famous? Let's start with what the existing evidence tells us about human nature.

Humans are all, for the most part, wired to be deceived (and, perhaps, exploited) by the dream of celebrity status. Understanding this cognitive predisposition can help to explain the durability of the search for celebrity, but it also offers insight that, I hope, will help us all to get on with our lives—whether we are seeking to be an *American Idol* finalist or trying to climb the corporate ladder. First off, people are, in general, pretty terrible at assessing their own abilities. College students are bad at guessing their own IQ (usually overestimating it, naturally) and numerous studies have shown that people overrate their creative talents. This has been called, not surprisingly, the *American Idol* effect. If you have ever watched the show, you have undoubtedly asked yourself, *How in the world does that person think he or she can sing? Is that person completely deluded?* I saw some of them warming up at my audition. Many were truly terrible, but they sang with a bizarre boldness that invited scorn from the other contestants, and they were oblivious of that too. In fact, the kind of squirm-inducing overconfidence that has helped to make shows like *American Idol* entertaining (in that enjoying-the-humiliation-of-others kind of way) may be perfectly natural.

A 2011 study published in the journal *Nature*, for example, suggests that overconfidence and the tendency to overestimate ability is a characteristic conferred on humans by evolution. While this exaggerated confidence can lead to crazy decisions (naked bungee jumping, anyone?) and even put individuals at risk, in the aggregate and over time it has provided us with an evolutionary advantage and, thus, has established a home in our DNA. The study found, for example, that if the evolutionary rewards (beating a competitor in a fight for food or a fine-looking mate) outweigh the risks (getting pummeled), then being overconfident is, from an evolutionary perspective, a good thing. But the authors of the study note that while overconfidence may have conferred an adaptive advantage in the distant past, it might not be as beneficial in the context of modern society (though it clearly helps the producers of reality TV). Like our evolutionarily determined desire for extra calories—a predisposition that was a big evolutionary advantage ten or twenty thousand years ago—the tendency toward overconfidence might not always work to our advantage now.

The inability to assess our own talent has been found in numerous domains, and even among the very young. A study of seventy-eight grade four students, for instance, found that the kids were, to quote the authors of the study, "remarkably poor predictors of their own creativity." Research on point has consistently found that self-reports about talent—whether about art, writing, science, math, singing or acting—tell us very little about actual, objectively assessed ability. So when Ryan Seacrest asks an *American Idol* contestant about his or her singing ability and the contestant responds that he or she is "awesome" and that "everyone thinks so," we can be fairly certain that he or she has no clue—a fact that the show uses to comic effect.

A closely related line of studies has found a strong tendency for people to rate themselves as above average. Indeed, if you believe the evidence, we all think we are pretty darn good at just about everything we do. A well-known 1981 study found that 93 percent of drivers think they are better than average. (From the perspective of my daily bike commute, I'd say that you are *all* seriously and chronically below average. I am, however, an awesome bike rider.) A US study of more than one million high school students found that 70 percent thought they had above-average leadership skills. Only 2 percent thought they were below average. Being highly educated apparently does not impact on self-knowledge. A whopping 94 percent of university professors think they are above-average teachers—which, by the way, I am. Just ask me.

People also believe they are more selfless, kind and generous than others and, to top it all off, better looking too. Research tells us that most people (particularly men) believe they are more attractive than average. Yes, as I noted early, celebrity culture often makes us feel dissatisfied with our appearance or a particular body part. But, for many of us, our built-in cognitive biases also delude us about our appearance. We are, it seems, dissatisfied but still aesthetically above average. Given the role of aesthetics in the celebrity universe, this is highly relevant to the present discussion. Research by Nicholas Epley and Erin Whitchurch, for example, has found that people are more likely to recognize an attractively enhanced picture of themselves than a less attractive picture (the yep-that-good-looking-person-in-the-picture-is-me! phenomenon). Another study, an online survey of more than twenty-six thousand Americans, found that most reckon they're above average in looks, giving themselves a 6 or 7 on a scale of 10. Among those under thirty, almost a third think they rank between an 8 and a 10!

While many psychological theories have been put forward to explain our tendency to rank ourselves as above average, recent work by Jonathan Brown from the University of Washington suggests that the primary driver is, quite simply, a desire to feel good about ourselves. In a series of experiments she found that people are particularly likely to rate themselves as better than average on traits that are viewed as socially important—that is, traits associated with character and skill, such as honesty or intelligence. He also found that the tendency increases when people have their self-worth threatened. In one of Brown's experiments he gave half the research participants an intelligence test that resulted in uniformly (fake) low scores. Those who received the insulting results were, when asked about their ability, more likely to rate themselves as better than average as compared to a control group that was not similarly insulted. Brown concluded that "people appraise themselves more positively than they appraise others because it makes them feel good about themselves to believe they are above average." But this and other research results also provide insight into what drives people who persist in pursuing celebrity status—namely their inability to realistically assess their own talent. And when their self-appraisal is challenged by, for example, those cruel *American Idol* judges, their response may be defensive and paradoxical. Instead of taking the advice of the experts and abandoning a singing career, unsuccessful contestants frequently storm out of the audition room, telling the world how great they are and how, one day, they'll be bigger than Michael Jackson.

Not surprisingly, this tendency also applies to how parents view their children. If you go on the perceptions of parents, every kid is above average. Every kid is special, smart and talented in some unique way. I've got four kids, so I know this tendency well. In fact, my kids seem to be well aware that I lack credibility. Recently I effusively praised my eldest daughter Alison's baking skills. Alison was unmoved. She looked steadily at me and said, "You are incapable of judging my baking. You are my dad." A good deal of research has shown that Alison is right (though I stand by my assessment of her lemon cake: it *is* first-class). Parents aren't terribly good at measuring how their kids stack up. Research has consistently shown that we overestimate our children's abilities in areas such as IQ, memory and language. An online survey, for example, found that 72 percent thought their kid was smarter than average. Only 6 percent thought their child was less intelligent than average. A 2009 study found that parents overestimated their kids' intelligence even more than the kids did. The study found that teachers were the most accurate predictors of a child's objectively measured intelligence. (Remember this the next time you feel like complaining to a teacher that he or she doesn't understand your child's unique gifts.) Another study, published in 2013, found that fully 91 percent of parents overestimated their children's emotional comprehension (the important social skill that, among other things, involves the understanding of the nature, cause and consequences of emotions and the ability to sense the emotional state of others).

In fact, parents aren't particularly adept at evaluating even the basic physical and mental condition of their children. For example, a 2012 study from the United States found that only 15 percent of parents think their kids are overweight, even though research has shown that about 32 percent of kids are overweight or obese. Similarly, parents underestimate the degree to which their children are unhappy or anxious and overestimate the degree to which they feel happy and satisfied.

We're Pollyannas too. In general, we are unrealistically optimistic about the future. This well-established psychological phenomenon, known in the literature as "unrealistic optimism" or "optimistic bias," has been found in innumerable studies. People tend, for example, to downplay the chance that bad things will happen to them. This is one reason why people knowingly do unhealthy and dangerous things. The thinking goes as follows: *Bad things happen to other people, not me! I won't get a nasty disease, so there's no need to wash my hands or quit smoking. I won't put on weight, so I don't need to watch my calorie intake or avoid junk food. And I won't get in a car crash, so there's no need to slow down or wear a seat belt. I know all those horrid things happen, but they are more likely to happen to someone else.* Note that the cognitive bias of unrealistic optimism also applies to positive outcomes. Most people overestimate the chances that their future will be bright, at least when asked to compare their chances to those of their peers. For example, studies have found that individuals overestimate the possibility of positive financial outcomes, that a cancer treatment will cure them or that they will achieve particular career goals. Since Neil Weinstein first described it in a famous 1980 experiment, this phenomenon has been demonstrated numerous times. Weinstein's study found that college students rate as better than their peers their chances of, among other things, getting a good job, living past eighty, having an achievement recognized in a newspaper and getting a career award. Since this 1980 study, some quibbling has occurred in the academic literature about the strength and source of the optimistic-bias tendency, but the research to date has been surprisingly consistent. We all think the future will turn out better for us than for the next guy. Again, this has obvious implications for our understanding of the ardor with which some people pursue celebrity status. *My chances of becoming a famous actor, musician or athlete are darn good, at least compared to you!* What I find most remarkable, however, is the degree to which optimistic sentiments persist, even when individuals are confronted with conflicting information. Even when they know the statistics that demonstrate how slim their chances are of becoming a celebrity musician, actor or athlete, they remain immovable. People think the statistics apply to other people, but not to them.

In 2011 neuroscientist Tali Sharot from University College London published a paper in *Nature Neuroscience* titled, appropriately, "How Unrealistic Optimism Is Maintained in the Face of Reality." Sharot found that the human brain is biologically wired to filter out information that does not confirm previously held optimistic beliefs. Sharot's team studied both the brain (using a special MRI machine) and behavior of research participants as they dealt with information that confirmed or conflicted with a previously held optimistic picture of the future. What they found was that humans selectively update knowledge and beliefs in a way that makes unrealistic optimism extremely resistant to change. Our brains let in and process the stuff that seems to support our unrealistic views while seeking to keep out all the negativity. As Sharot and her colleagues conclude, "Our brains and behavioral tendencies make us peculiarly susceptible to view the future through rose-colored glasses."

There are many specific examples of these biologically affixed rose-colored glasses operating in ways that directly support my supposition that unrealistic optimism plays an important role in the continuing desire to achieve celebrity status. I corresponded with Tali Sharot on this point and she agreed, saying the evidence tells us "people will continue believing in their dreams, even when faced with information that suggests it might not be a good idea."

An early paper with a particular focus on celebrity-oriented professions came to the same conclusion as Sharot. Those engaged in "artistic professions," the authors suggest, "are [the] most likely to succumb to this particular kind of over optimism." The authors note, for example, that girls training to be ballet dancers persist in their belief that they could have a professional career "even if explicitly confronted with the cruel facts, in particular that the rate of unemployment is extremely high and the income low." They found that the "girls dutifully listen to such information, [but] they are unshaken in their overoptimism believing that this may well be true but applies to the others." The authors also conclude that the same overestimation applies to would-be actors, which they cast as "one of the professions with the highest rate of unemployment in the whole labour force."

Studies also have shown that the optimistic tendency plays out in sport. A 2012 study from Germany, for example, followed almost 1600 elite-level soccer players between the ages of ten and twenty-three. The players all attended the training academies of the thirty-six German Bundesliga (the top tier) professional clubs. These academies are the primary source of professional soccer talent in Germany. So being asked to participate in one of these academies is a big deal—a sign you have true soccer talent. A majority of the players thought their chances of becoming a star were good. This belief endured despite the fact that it is well known that the chances of success are slim, even among this assemblage of tremendously talented and handpicked youths. How slim? Fewer than 5 percent of them will sign a professional contract, let alone have a significant, celebrity-worthy career. And yet, even though these young men could actually witness the rarity of success as they watched the vast majority of their older colleagues fail, they clung to their belief in their own glorious destiny. Indeed, the trend toward unrealistic optimism was remarkably strong in every age group. Even the older players in this study believed, on average, that their chances at success were good. This result surprised even the lead author of the soccer study, Verena Jung, from the Institute for Sports, Business & Society at EBS University in Germany. "I expected that the older they become, the more they would get realistic about the judgment of their chances," she told me. "But I found the opposite to be true."

The huge social profile of celebrities, the celebrity-making process and celebrity lifestyle add to the power of these cognitive biases. Celebrities are everywhere in popular culture, so it is not hard to find an example of a person who has "made it" by following a path similar to the one you are struggling on. I spoke to one actress who is no longer young by Hollywood standards (though she is young if measured against a normal-human standard), who continues to get a reasonable amount of work. She told me she remained hopeful about her chance for big success. As proof she pointed to several actors who made it late in life. "I am on my own path," she told me, "but just look at these other actresses who made it late in life! I know it can happen." Success stories exist that illustrate the possibility of triumph over almost every type of adversity. If you want to be a professional athlete but never got drafted by a professional team, there are many examples you can turn to for inspiration and "evidence"—albeit anecdotal in nature—that success is still possible. The almost-certain-to-be-in-the-Hall-of-Fame quarterback Kurt Warner, for example, was never drafted and had a job packing groceries before he landed a job with an NFL team. Now he is considered one of the best quarterbacks of all time. If you are no longer a teenager and still crave success as a pop star, you can look to Sheryl Crow—she was a near-ancient thirty-one years old when she first made it big. And if you do not conform to the Hollywood stereotype of beauty and thinness you can point to full-figured actresses like Melissa McCarthy and Queen Latifah.

The tendency to seek out and use information that confirms previously held beliefs is called confirmation bias and is, of course, closely related to the neurological and behavioral phenomenon covered above. Much has been written about this tendency in the context of politics. Conservatives see and seek out evidence that confirms their conservative beliefs, whether it is about gun control, taxation or gay marriage. Liberals do the same. When it comes to the topic of climate change, it has been demonstrated that individuals gravitate toward "evidence" that supports their worldview—no matter how crazy or marginal. Confirmation bias can affect personal decisions. And, I believe it plays a particularly salient role in how fame and celebrity are viewed as obtainable and desirable goals, either by individuals in relation to their own career choice or by parents in relation to their kids. Stories of success have huge sway. Indeed, research has shown that a single powerful anecdote can have more persuasive force than a mountain of statistics, and this seems particularly to be the case in the context of celebrities. Their stories of success fill magazines and other media, and when they are presented from the perspective of a wealthy actor, singer or athlete looking back on his or her life, they can appear to be compelling proof that a celebrity life is not that far out of reach.

SUNK COSTS AND NO PLAN B

Many of the people that I spoke with were neither naive nor young. On the contrary, many had been at the fame game for a long time. I spoke to actresses and actors in their mid-thirties and to full-time touring musicians who were well past the age at which many people are married and have families. They seemed to be well aware of the odds against their achieving real success and money. Nevertheless, they stuck with it. Why? Of course, many of them simply love the life and the artistic process. But numerous other forces add to the pressure to continue following your dream.

For example, research tells us the longer they stay in the game and appear to be taking steps toward success—managing not to get cut from a sports team, getting a callback for an acting job, performing at SXSW—the more likely they'll hang in. On some level, this may seem like a logical decision: after all, the aspiring stars are receiving positive feedback that suggests their chances at success are increasing. But, to believe this is to forget that the longer they pursue a dream job with a low chance of success, the more the opportunity costs increase—in terms of money, time and future career options. In other words, as one gets older (and for most of the fame-game professions, that is the mid-twenties), the risks intensify. So even if the chances of success go up (e.g., you've made it to a high-level sports team or got a small part on a TV show), so do the costs. One would think that this reality would cause people to reevaluate. But another cognitive bias, often called the escalation of commitment or the tendency to honor sunk costs, can kick in, making a career adjustment very difficult.

Cognitive bias applies even if we aren't succeeding at our chosen career. It happens even if, from an objective point of view, it appears that we are failing to achieve our stated goals. This is because the more we invest in a decision, whether in terms of money or time, the more likely we are to find ways to justify and rationalize the decision. It happens with gamblers (hold instead of fold). It happens with investors (buy instead of sell). It happens with married couples (counseling instead of divorce). And it happens with prime ministers and presidents (um ... war in Iraq).

For performing artists, another dimension to the escalation of commitment appears to exist, and that is the "No Plan B" phenomenon described to me by Ramesh and many other actors, musicians and artists. CJ, my guide to SXSW, felt it was important to go all in—to live the life of a musician. And another interviewee, a successful painter from New York, informed me that artists must think as the sixteenth-century Cortés did, when he landed in the New World to conquer the Aztecs: "Burn the ships. It is victory or death."

I asked TV and movie actor Bryan Greenberg about the No Plan B mentality. I wanted his view for two reasons. First, he has had a terrific career, with leads (e.g., *Prime*) and great parts (e.g., *Friends with Benefits*) in many Hollywood movies, and has starred in successful TV shows (e.g., *One Tree Hill* and *How to Make It in America*). I think it fair to say that he has achieved celebrity status. Second, and more importantly, he is the guy who gave my new friend Ramesh the No Plan B advice! "The reason I never had a plan B when pursuing my dreams is 2 fold," Greenberg told me in an email. "One: I wasn't good at anything else. And two: The path to success in my field is so challenging that I knew if I gave myself an out, I would take it. Humans always take the path of least resistance. So I just put side blinders on and trotted down one path."

It is a strategy that seems nearly suicidal, at least from a life-plan perspective. I asked Michael Simkins about it during our discussion in London. "Only an actor would understand this," he said. "It makes total sense. If you have a plan B, it can easily become plan A. You get used to the security and to the money associated with a real job. Suddenly plan B is plan A and, before you know it, you aren't acting anymore. If you get off the acting tightrope, it is hard to get back on." From the outside, those caught in the vortex of an escalation of commitment often seem irrational. But you can see how it can happen. When you have invested time, money and effort in a particular activity, it can be very difficult to walk away or cut your losses, even if, from an objective point of view, that is the more rational decision.

The trap caused by the escalation of commitment catches parents too. Increasingly, kids focus on one or two activities at a very young age. The costs and time investment can be significant. Hockey parents in Canada, for example, invest thousands of dollars in sticks, skates, power skating lessons, hockey camps, travel, etc. The authors of a recent book, *Selling the Dream*, found that it isn't unusual for families to sink more than $300,000 into a youngster's hockey career (imagine if that money was invested!). Parents may feel that given this commitment, they should keep going, even if junior isn't looking like the next Wayne Gretzky.

A friend and colleague, Camilla Knight, studies the role of parents in the experiences of children and adolescent athletes. Before her life as a researcher, Camilla was an elite tennis player. So it is no surprise that much of her research has focused on tennis parents. Over the course of her academic career—she is now a lecturer in sport psychology at Swansea University in the UK—Camilla has interviewed hundreds of parents. She has found that the motivations for putting kids into a particular sport are, of course, complex and varied, but that many do hope it will lead to a successful collegiate or professional career. "If they stop funding or supporting their children in the way they have previously," Camilla told me when I asked her about the problem of escalating commitment, "parents can feel that all their previous support has been for nothing.... In fact, one parent best described it to me as being like a hamster on a wheel and not being able to stop."

Camilla told me about another aspect to the sunk-cost dilemma, one that is unique to the situation of parental support: "Having committed so much already they find themselves in a difficult situation because they feel that suddenly stopping could prevent their children from succeeding ... or be viewed by their children as an indication that their parents no longer believe in them."

We have seen that we are biologically and cognitively set up to believe the celebrity life is both realistic and attainable. We are terrible at assessing our own abilities. We are neurologically constructed to be unrealistically optimistic about our future. We have a tendency to seek and use information that confirms our beliefs and ignore facts that conflict with those beliefs. And once we are on a particular career path, we may find it difficult to cut our losses. Adding to this near-perfect storm of cognitive tendencies is the fact that most of us are appallingly bad at using and comprehending probabilities. Indeed, we are not very good, in general, at thinking statistically, particularly when the relevant probabilities are extremely remote. When we hear, for example, that only eleven out of thirty thousand minor hockey players will play in the NHL, the numbers have very little persuasive force because—again, for most people— they just don't mean anything. People see the success of the few, well-publicized sport stars and this is what guides their perceptions of chance. Many parents likely think, *Hey, eleven*

kids made it! Or. *Well, my kid could be one of the eleven, I like them odds!*

This tendency to focus on the exciting numerator—the eleven who made it to the NHL—rather than the denominator—the thirty thousand who didn't—is an example of yet another bias in our thinking, often called denominator neglect. This tendency is particularly common when the numerator is high profile or easily imagined, which is exactly the situation with celebrity professions. Stories about the few individuals who make it in celebrity professions dominate our popular culture. They *are*, to a large degree, our popular culture. When you tell a parent that each year only twenty-five TV roles are up for grabs for the more than twenty thousand child actors, this disconcerting fact may have little impact on a parent's decisions because the ridiculously low probability simply does not register, especially if they are exposed to a well-known story of success that runs counter to the statistical reality. A *People* magazine cover story will always win out over a statistical analysis.

Not long ago the *Winnipeg Free Press* carried a story about the vast amount of money that hockey parents invest in the sport. A few sentences uttered by one of the parents the reporter interviewed serve as a powerful example of how the long odds can be known but still not resonate. "I'll guarantee you one thing," the hockey dad said, "If you don't buy a lottery ticket you can't win. That's why if parents can afford it, they will pay. It's an endless, hour-less [sic] debate but at the end of the day in order to keep up with the competition level, you have to train year-round.... Everybody says only one player will make it out of a million. Why can't it be yours?"

Of course, in this context, the lottery ticket is not a piece of paper purchased at a corner store for a few dollars, but a child's time, a family's resources and, perhaps for all of them, lost opportunities to experience other things.

CHAPTER 9

SIMON COWELL AND SOCIAL PRESSURE

"You can sing," Simon Cowell told Rachel Miller* after she finished a jazzy version of "Somewhere over the Rainbow." Cowell's praise was delivered in his now infamously snide and matter-of-fact tone. To the then seventeen-year-old Rachel, it didn't feel like much of a compliment. "I thought he was being sarcastic!" Rachel told me with a laugh as she reflected, eleven years later, on her *American Idol* experience.

Though she always dreamed of being a famous actor, she was often told she had a good voice, and not just by family members. So when the auditions for the first season of *American Idol* rolled through Chicago, a short trip from her hometown of Madison, she was encouraged by family and friends to give it a try. *American Idol* had not yet become the cultural phenomenon we know today and she saw participation as a bit of a lark and an opportunity to get more singing experience. At this point in her life she had already committed a lot of time and energy to acting and singing, mostly in musical theater. Fame and fortune was the

---

* This is not her real name. As you will see, given her current profession, publicizing her *Idol*-fueled search for celebrity is probably not a career-enhancing move.

objective. "I am from a lower-middle-class family. The fantasy, the ultimate goal, was high income. [Stardom] is portrayed like you will get millions."

Rachel also told me that she felt a lot of pressure—from family and from society generally—to follow her dreams and reach for the stars. To never give up. To strive for fame. To be her best. To never say never. These were the messages she got from everyone in her social sphere. "Not that it's bad or that I didn't appreciate the support from family and friends," she told me. "But all of the cards I got were 'follow your dream' cards."

We have seen how powerful individual psychological and, even, evolutionary predispositions exist that keep the celebrity dream alive. But, as Rachel's comments highlight, social and economic forces are also at play. This includes the Western world's love affair with ambition and the idea of "following your dreams." This love affair is relatively new. For most of human history ambition was viewed as either a vice or a sin. (For example, Shakespeare warned us in *Henry VIII*: "I charge thee, fling away ambition: By that sin fell the angels.") But over the past hundred years or so the mix of consumer culture and the rise of the American Dream ethos recast ambition as a virtue. It is tough to escape the reach-for-the-stars mentality. It is everywhere. Using an internet search tool (Google's Books Ngram Corpus, which gauges how frequently a phrase appears in the millions of English-language books published over decades to give an indication of linguistic and cultural trends) I traced the incidence of a range of phrases associated with chasing our celebrity dreams.* What did I find? Over the past sixty years we

---

* Thanks to Jean Twenge for suggesting this approach.

have been increasingly bombarded with phrases that tell us to never give up, to dream big and to reach for the stars. In fact, virtually every phrase that I could think of as an analog to the idea that we should "follow your dreams" has increased in use since 1950. That key phrase has increased in use by a factor of about 50. In other words, it is used fifty times more often now than it was in 1950. (To be honest, the phrase was almost *never* used in the 1950s, so my calculation is conservative.) "Never give up" has increased in use by a factor of 6.2. "Reach for the stars" by a factor of 27. "Dream big" by a factor of 21. "Believe in yourself" by a factor of 8.9. "Never say never" by a factor of 54. "Be your best" by a factor of 4.3. And "do not give up" by a factor of 3.7. By way of contrast, consider these words and phrases that have *decreased* in frequency over the past sixty years: sacrifice, appreciation, obligation, service, teacher, engineer, fine arts, public interest, public duty and economic equality.

Research by Yalda Uhls at UCLA found a similar trend when she analyzed the most popular TV shows aimed at teenagers. She set out to map the degree to which, among other things, the value of "fame seeking" was embraced by the main characters. The results are striking. Fame went from fifteenth place (last place on the list of values analyzed in the study) in 1967 to *first place* in 2007. The study, published in 2012, also found that the value of "achievement" rose from tenth place in 1967 to second in 2007, and the value of "community" fell from number 1 in 1967 to number 11 in 2007.

Of course, the relationship between popular culture and social values is complex. The media both reflects and shapes popular perceptions. But whether the popular representations referred to above are leading or reflecting public sentiment, it is hard to deny that a shift has occurred. In our current culture, the idea of bettering ourselves and seeking fame is framed as a noble endeavor, almost a social expectation. If you have a chance to make it celebrity big, that should be your central priority. Just think of all the heart-wrenching storylines from shows like *American Idol*, *The Voice* or *So You Think You Can Dance*, where a contestant must put individual dreams of fame above, say, staying with a dying parent or working at a job to put food on the table for a young family. The sacrifice for the (illusory) ticket to fame is presented (usually over a bit of sentimental-sounding pop music and with the requisite tears and hugs) as the right and honorable choice. The sacrifice for a shot at fame is what is expected of you.

(Quick side observation regarding *So You Think You Can Dance:* This is an entertaining show, but rich celebrity dancer? You have a better chance of being abducted by aliens and crowned the ruling monarch of Alpha Centauri.)

Rachel Miller's *Idol*-propelled search for fame continued past the audition phase, though she was soon to make a curious, and culturally antithetical, decision about her career. After a brief round of banter among the *Idol* judges, Paula Abdul announced, in a bubbly Paula Abdul manner, that Rachel had made it through to the next round. "Work on your stage presence," was Cowell's last bit of advice, halfheartedly lobbed in Rachel's direction as she was heading out of the room. At least that is how she remembers the otherworldly encounter. Months later, Rachel found herself in "Hollywood" (in the first year of *Idol*, the famous "Hollywood week" took place in Pasadena) for the next round. She didn't last long. Once again, the judges thought her stage presence was not *Idol*-esque. She was given the boot.

She told me the *Idol* experience was fun, a great opportunity and just as weird as you might expect. "Everyone was very nice and, yep, many of the contestants were there solely because they wanted to be famous," she said. But she wasn't overly concerned about not progressing. She had other plans, including competing at an event in New York sponsored by the International Modeling and Talent Association (IMTA).

IMTA is the largest modeling and performance conference in the world. It has also been called the most expensive. Convention participants can pay as much as $10,000 for an experience that is portrayed, mostly by IMTA, as a stepping-stone to superstardom. It is attended mainly by kids, teenagers and young adults desperate for fame and celebrity. And the organizers play to this constituency. IMTA, according to its website, "is the place where the world's top model and talent agents, managers and casting directors come to find new faces." It is also, for the vast majority, the place where young wannabe celebrities are separated from a significant amount of money for the privilege of, basically, hanging out with and competing against other wannabes.

The existence of entities like IMTA highlights the other force driving our social commitment to the celebrity dream: fostering and supporting the dream is a massive and profitable business. The celebrity industry, which includes dance classes, singing lessons, modeling conventions, online talent "agencies" and beauty pageants, exploits the fantasy of celebrity and all the cognitive predispositions and personal vulnerabilities that keep the fantasy alive. Indeed, from the perspective of this industry, the more the prospect of celebrity seems to be a tangible and reachable goal, the better. The industry has nothing to gain by telling celebrity aspirants the truth.

A significant portion of fame-oriented competitions, classes and services seem to be full-on scams. Do not let yourself or (more likely) your kids succumb. A modeling class, for example, cannot teach you to be tall, beautiful, photogenic and rail thin. That requires, in descending order of importance, genetics, genetics, genetics and, if genetics don't do it, a diet of water and lettuce. An open audition for a kid show that sounds too good to be true *is* too good to be true. These are swindles designed to hook families into spending ridiculous amounts of money for photos, representation, acting classes, etc., on the promise of a chance to appear on TV. The Disney Channel is often rolled out as a possible employer. Real TV shows don't need to hold open auditions in malls to find actors.

Unlike most of these exploitative ventures, IMTA appears to have helped a few current celebrities to achieve success. Indeed, what makes IMTA alluring is that many well-known actors and models are alumni of IMTA events, including Ashton Kutcher, Katie Holmes, Jessica Biel and Eva Longoria. Many of these stars give glowing testimonials on the IMTA website. Ms. Holmes, for example, gushes thus: "Let's just say, a girl from Toledo would never end up in a Hollywood movie if it weren't for the IMTA." (That kind of analysis of a personal career trajectory is undoubtedly distorted by another cognitive bias called hindsight bias. It is likely that when Ms. Holmes looks back through the lens of a successful—albeit a Tom-Cruise-tainted— career, it seems to her that IMTA played a significant role. Her assessment doesn't, obviously, include the sizable role played by luck. Nor does it include consideration of the thousands upon thousands of wannabes who took the same steps and never even got a nibble of interest.) While a handful of IMTA alumni have made it celebrity big—a fact that IMTA deploys to create a glamorous narrative to overwhelm the grim statistical reality—it is easy to find stories of heartbreak associated with participation in IMTA. An article in the *New York Observer* describes a young lady who shelled out more than $42,000 in her efforts to achieve celebrity through IMTA. "I didn't have tons of money before-hand, but the agency just told me to charge it to credit cards and that I would make it all back within a year when I was famous," she told the magazine.

I thought I should check out IMTA myself, but no one from the organization returned any of my emails. So, I dropped by the conference, uninvited.

The event is held in a large hotel in midtown Manhattan. As soon as I walk in the front door I see gaggles of young, attractive model-types. I am clearly in the right place. Moments later, half a dozen shirtless, well-built, twenty-something, unselfconscious men zip by, in a hurry to get to a place where shirtless men are urgently needed. I meander around the lobby chatting with participants. I meet a thirteen-year-old from Chicago ("I can act, sing and dance!"), a twenty-year-old from South Africa ("I hope to be a successful model"), two teenage boys from Canada ("We always wanted to be famous") and a seven-year-old who wants to be like Selena Gomez. It goes on and on. When I ask why they came to the IMTA event, almost all say they view it as a stepping-stone to stardom—often seeming to paraphrase IMTA promotional material—and several drop references to

Katie Holmes as evidence to support their decision (confirmation bias in action!). The seven-year-old used a crowd-sourcing website to raise the money necessary to attend IMTA. (I was told by most that the cost hovered around $5000, but no one would give me an exact figure.) Her website informs contributors that she needs to get to IMTA because it is her "biggest dream" and a "once in a lifetime experience," and her ultimate goal is "to be an actor with Disney Channel."

Numerous seminars are underway. I stroll down a hallway and stick my head in an open door. At the front of the hall sit two bored-looking men (I later find out they are moderately successful casting directors). The room is full of children and parents. A long queue of kids behind a microphone anxiously wait their turn to ask the two men for advice. They all ask some version of the same question: how do I become famous? And the answer is always the same: work hard, prepare and make the most of every opportunity. Just before I turn to leave, a little blond girl, who looks to be about seven or eight years old, gets on her tippy toes and asks, "How do you make a casting director remember you?"

One of the men smiles, leans into the microphone and says, "Well, darling, just be as cute are you are now." Sage advice.

A section of the conference floor is roped off. This is the competition area. It is the main ballroom and where the bulk of the participants seem to be located. I try several times to talk my way in. No luck. Finally, after a long chat with one of the conference "guards" (he looks more like a model than a bouncer) explaining my project, I get escorted inside, which is set up like a fashion show, with a well-lit runway and large video screens on either side. As I walk in, grade school boys are, one at a time, working the catwalk in the "jean competition." An announcer with a voice that has a beauty-pageant vibe calls out a four-digit number ("neeeext up ... five, threeee, nine, siiiiiiiix!") and a small boy wearing the designated number confidently marches down the runway with all the swagger of a high-end model who has done it a million times before.

I am standing behind the panel of judges who seem only half interested. They will grade the little models, and a few of the boys—a very few—will get a callback and the chance to do it again in front of agents, casting directors, etc. I have absolutely no idea what they are being graded on. How does one nine-year-old wear his jeans better than the next nine-year-old?

But what about our *Idol*-castoff, Rachel? How did IMTA treat her? Was the convention in New York an expensive, fruitless scramble for a grab-and-a-miss at the celebrity brass ring?

In fact, Rachel's experience at the IMTA event turned out to be the kind of anomaly that keeps the illusion of fame alive. Like the participants I spoke with, she also paid big. She told me that while she can't remember details, she believes her participation in the event cost around $2500, plus airfare and hotel. She also needed to pay for professional photos in order to produce a model-quality portfolio. This cost more than $1000. For a family that didn't have a lot of money, this was a significant investment. But, amazingly, her participation in the event *did* result in the promised meetings with well-established agents. She won or did well in all of the IMTA competitions she competed in, including the singing and modeling categories. And this led to a contract with a respected talent agency with offices in New York and LA. Next up for Rachel, a move to LA and work with a hit-generating music producer who has written or produced songs for the likes of Céline Dion, Kylie Minogue and Eminem. Rachel's dreams of fame and fortune nudged significantly closer. *This is really going to happen*, the seventeen-year-old thought. *I am going to be a star.*

PLEASE NOTE: PUNCTUALITY IS EXTREMELY IMPORTANT!

If you spend any amount of time online researching the concept of "celebrity," one thing quickly becomes clear: a lot of companies are out there ready to help you become famous. There are, for example, StarNow ("where talent gets discovered—actors, models, musicians wanted … no experience required"!), Casting Now ("a platform to showcase your talent"), Click My Talent ("a talent profile service") and One Source Talent (OST). The last one is ubiquitous. Indeed, many other online celebrity career services funnel you back to One Source Talent. A modeling database called Model Search America, which says it will "see you at the top," has an "apply now" link after the question "Do you want to be a model or an actor?" The "apply now" link takes you to One Source Talent. The exact function of OST is unclear, but the flashy website, which prominently displays the company tagline "No more what ifs," makes it appear that a career as a model or actor is both common and easily obtained. The homepage displays a picture of a teenage girl (most of these celebrity-focused companies seem to be aimed at tweens and teenagers) with an invitation to "Become a Model/Actor" written next to her smiling face.

Sounds good! I decide to sign up.

I click on the "apply" link. This takes me to a registration page that starts with the question "Are you ready to take your shot?" In addition to my views on "shot taking," they want my name, date of birth, email address and phone number. That's it. I also upload a picture of my old, less-than-celebrity-like face. I push the submit button and, no exaggeration here, I *instantaneously* get a call. I swear it came so fast that I had to lift my hand from the mouse that just clicked "send" to my cell phone that told me a call was coming from New York.

"Um … hello?"

"Hi! This is One Source Talent!"

"Wow! You guys are fast. No fooling around!" I respond.

"Well, you know what this call is about!" replies the friendly and enthusiastic-sounding woman. "We are having an assessment here in New York in a few days. Would love for you to come by."

I agree that it sounds like a great opportunity, even though I have no idea what an "assessment" is.

More than anything, these online "services" (I use that term loosely) appear to be a way to exploit the desire for a glamorous career by promising to get you exposure with casting directors and modeling agents. These companies refer to a range of jobs in the entertainment industry, though their connection to these jobs is unclear. It seems likely they simply want their clients to believe a link exists and that thousands of jobs are in fact available. The Model Search America website, for example, tells us that there are "all kinds of opportunities out there" with "the millions of TV networks" that "need content to fill air time." This remarkable claim is followed a few sentences later by this: there "are thousands of networks out there too" (what happened to the millions?), including "Disney, Fox, CBS, NBC, ABC, ESPN, VH1, MTV, FX, Comedy Central, Discovery Channel, Food Network, Spike, TNT, Sprout, Nick Jr., E entertainment and the list goes on and on." The webpage concludes thus: "If you want to be on these networks you have to start somewhere and that is why Model Search America is here for you."

"I'm looking forward to my meeting," I tell Jennie, my new personal contact at One Source Talent. She tells me that I don't need to bring anything to the assessment. No special clothes. No prepared bit of acting that they can use to "assess." And no special photos or acting résumé. But, I suspect, a credit card might be needed.

I decide to get my assessment at One Source Talent's Hollywood office. That way, when I get signed to work on a big studio movie, I won't have far to go. A few days before my appointment I get an email from OST. I am told to "dress to impress." That "punctuality is extremely important. Do not just be on time; be early!" And to "relax, be yourself and professional. When your opportunity comes to shine, stand out with a positive attitude and professional behavior."

I arrive at OST early. How could I not? An attractive young receptionist in the slick-looking office greets me. A framed magazine cover behind her tells me that OST was, in 2008, one of the country's fastest growing companies. About twenty people are in the room, with appointments at the same time as me. Most are young children with their parents. The latter primp and fuss over their aspiring little celebs: there is much anxious pacing, hair spraying, combing and parental injunctions to *stand up straight.* It all got me a bit nervous. Perhaps I was a tad unprepared. A young man wearing a bowler hat (and a smile that, I think, had a wisp of irony attached to its edges) called out my name and invited me to get in line for a picture, which, another pretty young woman told me, was "purely for our records." Beside me was a boy who appeared to be about five years old. He was wearing a flashy outfit that looked like a little version of a tux you might wear on a Vegas stage circa 1970. His name was Sparkle. "Just Sparkle,"* he said confidently to one of the OST staff. Sparkle was called in for his assessment before me. As he disappeared into an office I heard a female voice say something like, "Hi, Sparkle, I am the head of West Coast youth talent identification." About ten minutes later it is my turn. Pretty young woman number three invites me into a small office. She tells me to stand in front of her desk for the "audition." Not an assessment, but an audition. Gulp. *Are they going to ask me to act?*

"So what are your career ambitions?" she asks.

"Nothing too grand. I am always looking for new experiences," I reply ambiguously.

"Do you have any experience?"

"Actually, I was the lead singer for a rock band," I say, keeping it truthful, but leaving out any reference to the relevant decade.

She then asks me about my day job ("I have flexible hours"), whether I would be ready to work soon ("Sure!") and whether I have professional photos. I respond with a "yes" to this question; I had them done for my last book. She informs me that I will

---

* He actually had a different, but very similar, one-name name.

probably need new ones, even though she has no idea what my old ones look like.

"Well, you have a great look." I do not. "You are perfect for something we have coming up next week," she says. "Be ready for a call! Thanks and goodbye."

That was it. No singing. No acting. No posing. I interacted with OTS staff for a total of about two minutes, and that included asking pretty-young-woman number one to order me a taxi. I didn't have much of an opportunity to shine, stand out or display my positive attitude and professional behavior.

I wonder how much time Sparkle got.

Months pass and I never get the call. Apparently my look isn't *that* great. I do, however, continue to receive regular emails from One Source Talent asking me to come in for an "assessment." Clearly I did not "shine" or "stand out" enough for them to remember that I have already had one.

CHAPTER 10

LUCK, "IT" AND TEN THOUSAND HOURS

"One thing people don't understand is that there is so much luck involved." This reality dawned on Rachel after just a few weeks in LA. "I am not a great singer," she told me with a laugh. "I'm good. But I got lucky. Luck got me to LA. There are so many talented girls. So many! I was in the right place at the right time. You need so much luck to get anywhere."

Luck plays a significant role in every career, of course. The adage about being "in the right place at the right time" could apply to almost any profession, from accounting and teaching to playing quarterback for the New England Patriots. ("Dear Drew Bledsoe, Thank you for getting injured. Love, Tom Brady.") But because of the huge number of people scrambling for a very small number of fame-creating positions, and because the public, casting directors, music producers and the market are all fickle, luck plays a particularly significant role in the realm of celebrity. Also, unlike, say, being a track-and-field champion, success at a celebrity job depends on a great deal of subjective assessment—an assessment that can be influenced by a boatload of uncontrollable factors (did the casting director have enough coffee before you walked into the room?). As of this writing, Usain Bolt is the fastest man alive. Period. Who is the best actor or singer or, even, quarterback? (Okay, the last one is obviously Tom Brady, but some may disagree. They would be wrong, but other, less-informed, opinions exist.)

Many of the actors and musicians I spoke with shared Rachel's appreciation of the massive role of luck, especially those who had enjoyed a degree of success. Michael Simkins put it this way: "Luck is more important than talent. Theoretically, you can get by without talent. Talentless actors make it. But without luck, you are fucked." This view is also held by the stratospherically successful, or at least that is what I have been told by a reliable source. Tim Monich is a renowned acting coach. He taught at Juilliard in New York for years and now works closely with the biggest stars on planet Earth, including Brad Pitt, Tom Cruise, Leonardo DiCaprio, Cate Blanchett, Nicole Kidman, Matt Damon, Clive Owen and Juliette Binoche, to name but a few. Monich was in Vancouver working with Owen and Binoche when we met up in a downtown coffee shop. He told me emphatically that every star he works with—all of them— realizes how lucky they are. "Leo and Brad? [*Leo* and *Brad* … love it.] Yes, they are ridiculously good-looking and talented. They work very hard. But they *know* how lucky they are. All are very aware that they have won the lottery."

The philosopher Seneca said, "Luck is what happens when preparation meets opportunity." This quote, a go-to axiom for motivational speakers, football coaches, advice columnists and inspirational kitty posters is, with all due respect to the dead Roman, wrong. Luck happens to those who are lucky. Period. And, please remember, the distribution of luck is random. That is why it is called luck. You can't do anything to enhance your luck.

Despite the honest calculation of the role played by luck in the careers of the artists I interviewed, a calculation that apparently resonates with seriously lucky Leo and Brad, many of us often greatly overestimate the degree to which we can control the uncontrollable. We imagine, for example, that our thoughts and actions can have an impact on outcomes that are entirely or largely beyond our control. This phenomenon, known as the illusion of control, operates in a range of contexts, including gambling, investing and the management of health risks. And like many of the other relevant psychological traits (unrealistic optimism, overconfidence, optimistic bias) it seems to have a biological foundation, a proposition confirmed by recent brain-scan research. This is because appreciating causal connections—seeing a relationship between actions and getting food or avoiding a predator, for example—conferred an evolutionary advantage. As such, we err on the side of seeing a connection, even when one isn't there. And because we see a connection between a particular action and a particular outcome, we think our actions can have tangible impact. We are, in short, wired to believe we can control the uncontrollable.

Adding to this illusion is the fact that most people believe that celebrities have, to some degree, earned their status. It wasn't luck but skill and hard work that led to their fame and fortune. The survey of 650 American teenagers cited in a previous chapter, for example, asked them to consider why celebrities became successful. "Hard work" was selected more often than all the other options combined, including luck and innate talent. Why is this relevant? Even though we are constantly told, "If we can dream it, then we can achieve it," dreaming and achievement are, in fact, usually only tenuously connected. It is an illusion that one leads directly to the other. The talent pool is so massive and the assessment criteria are so complex and ambiguous, to say nothing of factors such as timing and genetics, that landing a celebrity job is probably 90 percent luck. Yes, for many jobs, particularly in the sports realm, you need to have the requisite talent and training to hold a ticket in the lottery, but luck still looms large. To paraphrase the Nobel Prize–winning psychologist Daniel Kahneman, career success is the result of talent plus luck. Great success (i.e., celebrity-sized success) is the result of a wee bit more talent and an incomprehensible amount of luck.

To make matters even more confusing, in some celebrity professions the nature of the needed "talent" is so mysterious and unquantifiable as to be beyond understanding, let alone control. This is the elusive "it" factor, the quality of cool that puts an artist a step ahead of the prevailing musical, theatrical, aesthetic, etc., zeitgeist.

It is, I humbly submit, nearly impossible to identify or manufacture the next "it" quality. Executives at Decca Records turned down The Beatles, famously predicting that "guitar groups are on the way out" and "The Beatles have no future in show business." Elvis was advised to stay in truck driving because he would "never make it as a singer." Yes, some people, such as Malcolm McLaren and his creation, the Sex Pistols, have successfully divined (or, through the lens of hindsight bias, they *seem* to have divined) cultural trends. But this kind of pop culture premonition is rare. If it could be done in a consistent manner, someone would be doing it. And if they were doing it, the "it" factor would be normalized, and then it wouldn't be an "it" quality anymore (one of the great pop culture paradoxes!). But this doesn't stop artists and the entertainment industry from trying.

For the music industry, finding or manufacturing "it" lies at the core of the business plan. I saw the phenomenon in spades at the SXSW convention in Austin. Indeed, for me, the overt attempt to project a cool image, which is, let's be honest, nothing more than a plea to the universe to recognize that "it" resides within the projector, was one of the most memorable and disheartening aspects of SXSW. It is a bit like that cliché about not wanting to see how sausages are made. I am a huge music fan, but seeing artists scramble for a piece of the music industry pie made me like the whole supposedly corporate-free and integrity-focused indie music scene a wee bit less. The constant posing was annoying. By posing, I mean the carefully curated social angst, the orchestrated I-am-on-the-fringes-of-society wackiness and the feigned disinterest, as if the musicians really had someplace better to be. It was all a serious turnoff. I am fully aware that few musicians are consciously adopting a pose that is meant to look like a pose. Indeed, looking like you aren't posing is one of the most important elements of successful posing, unless, of course, you are doing it ironically, in which case you must adopt a pose that projects a knowing pose-ness, but is still, at its core, authentic and anti-posing. It must be exhausting. The posing problem is most problematic onstage, though it is almost as annoying when you see bands strutting on the street or hanging after the show.

(By the way, I am fairly certain that I found this element of the image-manufacturing process irritating because it reminded me of my own sad rock-star ambitions and my own history of cringe-worthy posing. I had it all: the angst, the zany stage antics, the thrift-shop clothes, the pretended apathy and the Flock-of-Seagulls hair. As I said, cringe.)

The point I am trying to make is that you can't, through hard work, practice, posing or positive thinking, create the "it" quality that will vault you to celebrity status. It is largely luck—luck you were either born with, stumbled upon or were asked to join. (And the winner is: Ringo Starr!) Am I being too harsh? Bands that have very little hard-work-enhanced musical proficiency populate the best bands in history lists. *Rolling Stone* magazine puts The Ramones as the twenty-sixth greatest artists of all time. The Sex Pistols are listed at sixtieth. My personal favorite, The Clash, are ranked twenty-eighth. Those three bands are almost *all* "it" factor. Iconography is as important as the music. Ditto early Rolling Stones. Mick Jagger? Nothing but "it." I am currently a better guitar player than Joe Strummer was when The Clash made it big, and I am pretty bad. But Joe had more "it," in my humble opinion, than almost anyone on Earth.

At least some evidence indicates that the quality of a song has little to do with whether it will be a hit. In addition to the role of marketing, timing and "it," an element of randomness is involved in determining what becomes popular. Sociologists Matthew Salganik and Duncan Watts, in a 2008 study, found that perceptions of success seem to influence purchasing decisions more than quality. They created a list of songs and allowed approximately thirty thousand individuals to download their favorites, which resulted in a ranked list. They then inverted the list, so that the least popular songs were now ranked as the most popular, and invited another group to download their favorites. As predicted by the authors, the songs that were deemed unpopular in the first round were now popular. While some of the "best" songs rebounded, a clear self-fulfilling-prophecy effect was at work. Songs viewed as popular, become popular. In other words, the cream does not always rise to the top. Momentum, which the authors call "cumulative advantage," and luck ruled.

I am not arguing that talent and hard work are irrelevant. On the contrary, for most celebrity jobs, you need both to simply enter in the lottery. Talent and hard work are often—but not always—the baseline prerequisites. I am suggesting that, for most celebrity-oriented careers, you also need a huge amount of luck, a factor that is totally out of your control. Realizing this injects an important reality check into the discussion. You can't plan on and work toward being lucky. And you can't plan on or work toward becoming a celebrity. To suggest otherwise, as implied by our society's obsession with the idea of "reaching for the stars," is to promulgate a lie.

Think I am being too harsh? J.K. Rowling stands as another great illustration of the degree to which luck plays a role in the context of celebrity professions or, really, *any* profession. She has sold approximately 450 million books, making her one of the bestselling authors in human history. The eight Harry Potter movies form, according to some estimates, the largest-grossing film franchise ever. Now, given this status, and her millions of admiring fans, surely it was hard work and raw talent that propelled her to fame? Doubtful. Once again, luck had to be involved. And Rowling provides us with a bit of evidence.

In 2013 she wrote a crime novel, *The Cuckoo's Calling*, under a pseudonym, Robert Galbraith. The result? Some publishers turned it down. One of these now red-faced publishers has since admitted that she thought the manuscript was not unique, lacked a clear selling point and "didn't stand out." When it finally did get published, it received solid reviews but sold fewer than five hundred copies. Keep in mind that Rowling already had a literary agent, which is one of the first and biggest hurdles in the writing world. If she hadn't had an agent, the manuscript might not even have been considered for publication. My guess is it never would have been published at all.

When it was revealed that Rowling was the author, the book instantly became a bestseller, making this a rare real-world experiment illustration of the random nature of success. Duncan Watts, one of the authors of the song study noted above, commented that the Rowling book controversy demonstrated "that quality and success are even more unrelated than we found in our experiment." And "it is also clear that being good, or even excellent, isn't enough."

But what about sport celebrities? Success in the domain of sports isn't haphazard or arbitrary. The most talented and hardworking succeed. Right?

In fact, research tells us that, for most sports, success appears to be the result of a relatively random process that is, once again, influenced by luck and other factors that are out of our control. Some "measurable" performance-oriented sports, such as, say, sprinting, depend less on luck and rather more on talent, but luck is still involved. The element of luck begins with the genetic characteristics your parents "decide" to provide. And then your genetic gifts must be recognized and nurtured. After all, someone out there may exist who's even faster than Usain Bolt but doesn't know what he's got. As for the big professional sports—football, basketball, baseball, hockey, soccer, etc.—it is shockingly difficult to predict who is going to succeed. Even if an NHL team drafts a player—in itself a rare occurrence—the odds are that the draftee will not play in the NHL. Ditto the NFL. And if you don't get picked up relatively soon after the draft process is over, the chance of ever getting picked up diminishes rapidly.

Evidence of this kind of randomness appears in other sports too. For NFL quarterbacks—an absolutely *massive* financial investment for the owner of a team, so you know that the quarterback-assessment experts are doing everything within their power to get the selection process right—a careful historical analysis found that the relationship between actual performance and draft position is weak. In other words, despite analyzing mountains of player performance data, dissecting hours of video of quarterback candidates, watching quarterbacks run through a range of assessment exercises, and despite the fact that tens of millions of dollars are at stake, experts still don't know how to predict success. Indeed, studies have found that outside the first-draft round, the relationship between how high a player is drafted and that athlete's actual playing time is not particularly strong. This is true for all of the major professional sports. And the fact that athletes drafted in the first round play more frequently than others may be due more to concerns about "sunk costs" than actual talent. That is to say, teams may tend to play the guys in whom they've invested the most cash.

These findings about the rather arbitrary nature of the draft system and the difficulty of measuring and predicting success in professional sports are important from the perspective of this book because they highlight the somewhat ad hoc nature of making it as a professional athlete. Obviously you must possess otherworldly physical talent even to be in the mix. But you also must be the right player, in the right place, at the right time. In other words, even if you are handed the perfect genes and have the best parental and coaching support, an obsessive drive and an incredible work ethic, to make it as a professional athlete, much depends on blind luck.

While being really good at something—singing, guitar, dancing, acting, hockey, football, etc.—is absolutely no guarantee of fame and fortune, the question remains: how does a person become celebrity great at something? Can you work and dream and "never say never" your way to greatness in preparation for a run at fame?

Malcolm Gladwell's bestselling book *Outliers* made the ten thousand hours rule famous. The premise is that almost anyone can achieve greatness at an activity—golf, tennis, chess, violin, guitar, etc.—if they put in enough time. And "enough time," so the theory goes, is ten thousand hours. This jibes with the idea that hard work, persistence and following your dream will inevitably lead to success. It provides us with a sense of control over our future and a way to combat the notion that all is not, in fact, subject to luck and innate talent.

It's an interesting theory and it appeals to my egalitarian sensibilities. But the data are far from conclusive and, I think it is fair to say, suggests that the ten thousand hours theory is, at best, only part of the story. Indeed, for some activities, particularly in the area of sports, it is obviously wrong, or, at least, incomplete. I could train for twenty thousand hours and never run a fast marathon or be a great pitcher or a world-class golfer. A great deal of sport aptitude is dependent on innate ability largely determined by your biological, and particularly your genetic, makeup. A 2012 study published in the *British Journal of Sports Medicine* sought to tease out the relative contributions of genes and training in the development of an athlete. The authors conclude: "Although deliberate training and other environmental factors are critical for elite performance, they cannot by themselves produce an elite athlete." For that, you need a whole bunch of luck in the genetic lottery.

But what about pursuits such as music that appear to be less constrained by physical abilities? (Acting and modeling also are, to a large degree, constrained by your gene-determined looks, so I'd put these two celebrity activities in the same category as sports.) Can a musician practice her way to greatness? Not likely. Research by Zach Hambrick and colleagues explored the degree to which the amount of practice predicted the ranking of musicians. They found that practice accounted for 30 percent of the variance in the rankings. To quote the conclusion from their 2013 paper: "Deliberate practice is not sufficient to explain individual differences in performance." In other words, more than two thirds of an individual's ranking as a musician is determined by factors other than practice—and, more than anything, that other stuff is likely innate ability.

"Many want to believe that if you are sufficiently motivated anyone can become an expert at something," Zach Hambrick, a professor of psychology at Michigan State University, told me. "But the data simply do not support this position." He feels that the ten thousand hours idea endures because it fits so well with both democratic ideals and the anyone-can-make-it ethos of the American Dream. It fits with the dream of celebrity. "While it may be a nice idea," Zach says, "it just isn't true." Or, as perfectly encapsulated in the title of an article he wrote for *The New York Times*: "Sorry Strivers, Talent Matters."

I am not a genetic determinist. I do not, for example, think that we will be able to develop a test that will inform wannabes if they have the right genetic makeup for a particular celebrity profession. The roles played by genes in the context of human behavior are just too complex. Nor do I think we should let our genes constrain or dictate our future. If you are a short, slow man and want to play point guard, go for it. But know that ten thousand hours of hard work will not overcome the short, slow stuff. I have played guitar for more than ten thousand hours, probably closer to fifteen thousand. Seriously. I love it. And I am brutal. Terrible. I seem to be incapable of improving. It is as if I were stuck in a rut of mediocrity. Most of us are. That's why it is called mediocrity.

Even Sir Paul McCartney, whose success Gladwell explicitly attributes to the ten thousand hours rule, questions the theory. "I mean there are a lot of bands that were out in Hamburg who put in 10,000 hours and didn't make it, so it's not a cast-iron theory," McCartney said. He thinks that most groups that are successful put in a huge amount of work, but, he says, "I don't think it's a rule that if you do that amount of work, you're going to be as successful as the Beatles." Indeed. And the reverse is also true. Many successful bands had far fewer than ten thousand hours behind them when they signed a contract. As noted, many bands have been signed despite a lack of musical proficiency. It is often said that U2, one of the most successful bands in rock history, started writing songs because they couldn't play covers well enough.

It is obvious that the genetic lottery, and many other forces outside our control, combine to create innate ability. They all have a huge impact on our chances of fame-generating greatness. And this is just another way that luck reigns over our celebrity aspirations.

LUCKY RACHEL

So, how did luck play out for Rachel? Did it propel her to a celebrity career? In fact, luck did quite the opposite, and she couldn't be happier.

Before she left for Los Angeles, Rachel applied to and was accepted by the University of Wisconsin. But at this point in her young life, she was still committed to a career in the entertainment industry, so college was a backup plan (yep, her Plan B!). Still, she thought it couldn't hurt to attend the freshman orientation event before she made her big move to the West Coast. Seated across from her in a huge university hall, as the usually gregarious Rachel explains, was "the first man I couldn't talk to. I was totally tongue-tied." As luck would have it, that man was her future husband.

Her experience in LA played out as one might expect, though it was hardly glamorous. She moved into a small place with another girl who was also seeking fame and fortune. She met regularly with her producer and other musicians to write and strategize. And she was pushed to change her look. Many, for example, told the model-contest-winning Rachel that she needed to lose a few pounds—and her name. At the time, the pop-punk Avril Lavigne was big. Scrambling to find the "it" factor by capitalizing on the Avril wave, it was (pathetically) suggested that her new name should have some of the same Avril edge. The moniker "Madison Tyler"—the first name was a reference to her hometown—was selected. Naturally, she would also be expected to change her sound to fit the name. No jazzy interpretations for Madison Tyler.

She was offered a contract, but the whole thing didn't feel right. "I would have been creating a pop album for money and fame," she said. "Those are the wrong reasons." She felt this way even though fame and fortune had been for her, from a young age, the whole point. But when she saw it laid out in front of her, it no longer seemed attractive. And, perhaps most importantly, she couldn't stop thinking about that man. "So I told them thanks, but no thanks," Rachel told me. "They looked shocked. I don't think they had ever had someone turn down a contract."

Rachel headed home to Wisconsin. She got great marks and became the first person in her family to graduate from college. She went to law school. She became a lawyer for the federal government. And, of course, she got married to that man. Many of her friends didn't and still don't understand her decision. "Even my parents," Rachel tells me, "bless their hearts, because they were incredibly supportive during this whole process, were frustrated that I walked away." Everyone kept asking her why she would give up on her dream. You aren't supposed to stop reaching for the stars, especially when they are within your grasp.

But that isn't Rachel's view. "Saying no to that contract was the best decision I ever made." Not a hint of regret.

Rachel has never sung professionally since that time. Occasionally, she will do some karaoke. "It is fun to shock people!" she told me with a laugh. One night in 2008 she did just that. On a whim, she jumped onstage to sing karaoke in front of a local band. A reporter caught the performance and was impressed. He noted that the "slim, pretty Rachel" would "look good on a CD cover" and might be just the kind of singer that could catapult the band "into international superstardom."

REALITY TV AND YOUTUBE

Many individuals, including people in the entertainment business, suggested to me that it was now easy to become famous because of social media and reality TV shows. This may *seem* to be true. There are a lot of these shows around. And they offer a way to move rapidly up the fame food chain. During my travels and research for this book, it seemed as though I heard the name "Kim Kardashian" almost every day. She certainly shows up in *People* magazine a lot; she was in nearly every issue I read over the past year.

But the impression is misleading. It is still incredibly rare, as we have seen with *American Idol*, for individuals to become celebrity big through reality TV. While I could not find any systematically collected stats, the number of individuals who have gained big-time celebrity through a reality show remains small. Indeed, one could argue that the phenomenon of reality TV, with its emphasis on the desirability of stardom, has drawn more individuals into the fame-seeking game, thus increasing the denominator, and, as a result, making true celebrity status even more unlikely. The number of people playing the lottery has increased.

The same can be said of YouTube. Sure, many individuals have gained notoriety by posting videos on the site (okay, a select few have become *huge*, such as Justin Bieber), the number of popular YouTube-focused performers (often called YouTubers) is ever-increasing, and some have used the site to build on an existing career (e.g., Psy via the YouTube hit "Gangnam Style"). But until relatively recently few built a career solely on YouTube to the point where they have broad name recognition and substantial wealth. How many YouTube celebrities can you name, not including Bieber and Grumpy Cat? (Note: This question is *not* for the current crop of teenagers. If you believe recent research, many teenagers can name dozens of YouTubers and often rank them as their favorite performers, above Hollywood actors and conventional pop stars.) Then think of the tens of thousands of videos that exist. Do the math. You can make money from YouTube (advertising revenue is shared), but unless you get millions of views, the income is insignificant—between $0.80 and $6 for a thousand views. With approximately one hundred hours of content being uploaded *each minute*, the chance of standing out is astronomically slim. Again, while quality plays a role, luck is obviously a big, big factor.

I am not denying the rising power of social media, or the way it can facilitate the creation of artistic communities, or even satisfy elements of the desire for fame. Much has been written, for example, about the rise of the "micro-celebrity," which involves individuals building and playing to a relatively small audience. But in the search for mainstream, big-time celebrity status, YouTube, and for that matter Facebook, Instagram and Twitter, have emerged more as an expected part of a wanna-be's reach-for-the-stars fame-generating portfolio than a magical vehicle to instant fame. They are powerful new tools, but that's all. And as with reality TV, social media increases the number of individuals seeking celebrity—expanding the already enormous denominator—by making it easier for more and more to play the fame game.

Another theme I heard expressed was about the conflation of fame, success and talent. Indeed, the actor Olivia Munn picks it as her number-one issue. "The worst part about fame," she says, "is that some people confuse fame for success." What she and others are concerned about is the ability of social media and reality TV to propel people to a kind of talent-free fame. "But just because people want your picture or know your name doesn't mean you have success," Munn says.

"Andy Warhol would have loved it," longtime publicist Susan Blond tells me of the current wave of people who are famous for simply being famous. "Kim Kardashian? Warhol would have loved her. She's fun. She's kitsch." Blond should know. She worked with Warhol. She also worked with The Clash. The first thing I notice in her New York office is a framed gold record for The Clash's seminal album *London Calling*, my all-time favorite. Seeing it there gives me goose bumps. Blond was in several of Warhol's films, including the black comedy *Bad*, in which her character throws a screaming baby out the window. The scene is still hard to watch. She also worked with Britney Spears and Ozzy Osborne. Blond is just as engaging, opinionated and fun as you would hope someone with her eclectic background in the entertainment industry would be. She inspired the character of publicist Bobbi Flekman in the movie *Spinal Tap* ("Money talks, and bullshit walks!"), but has none of her edge. Thank goodness.

"Well, you might say they earned it. Some had sex on video" is her joking response when I ask if reality stars have earned their celebrity status. Blond seems to view the famous-for-being-famous phenomenon more as a critique of popular culture than as some kind of irritatingly unjust achievement. As Bobbi Flekman might say, it's all bullshit, why split hairs? "To be honest, it is hard not to be jealous of the people who have figured how to make money off of just their celebrity status. They get paid a huge amount just to go to parties," Blond says. Paris Hilton reportedly made around half a million for simply showing up at events. This phenomenon has helped to promote the idea that fame, and not the fostering of exceptional artistic talent, is a reasonable goal all on its own. This is why, I suppose, some kids say they want to be famous and not, for example, a great guitar player or an exceptional actor.

Blond is quick to dismiss those in the industry who claim to be above the drive for celebrity status. "Make no mistake, many great artists love the idea of fame. And I like celebrity. I like fame," Blond says. "But I get more excited about raw talent."

SO WHAT?

In this section of the book, I have touched on a few of the myriad reasons it is nearly impossible achieve true celebrity. In many ways, our entire social economy creates a massive pop culture–fueled positive-feedback loop that builds the illusion that celebrity status is both an attainable and a reasonable goal. And this illusion is kept alive by and plays to our biologically determined cognitive biases, which make us all susceptible to the belief that we can and should "reach for the stars" and "never say never." You may be thinking, so what? What does it matter that the illusion of celebrity-sized success shapes the hopes and ambitions of kids, families, struggling artists and many others besides? The answer is simple. If we can see through the illusion, then we can make better-informed decisions. And being aware of our cognitive biases allows us to be more sensitive to our actual strengths and weaknesses. This awareness will, I hope, allow us all to avoid celebrity-dream scams. Potentially, it will keep us from committing large amounts of personal and family resources to an unattainable goal. This is both a philosophical issue (do we really want a society where celebrity status is a primary goal?) and a practical challenge with real consequences. For example, a 2008 study of UK teachers revealed a growing concern about the impact of celebrity culture on the education environment because, as one teacher said, "pupils believe celebrity status is available to everyone" and "[students] do not think it is important to be actively engaged in school work as education is not needed for a celebrity status." Another noted that "[the students] believe that they are much more likely to achieve financial well-being through celebrity."

More broadly, the fact that so much of the modern world's social capital—in terms of time, cultural space and economic investment—is geared toward selling and seeking a goal that is, for all practical purposes, nonexistent should give us pause. The American Dream is based on the idea that if you work hard enough you can have a good life and do whatever you want. But the whatever-you-want carrot that is meant to drive our society forward does not—again, in any real sense—exist. The carrot at the end of the stick isn't real.

On a more personal level, the realization that the chance of making it celebrity big is so remote and so dependent on factors that are completely out of our control is liberating. Accepting that fact frees us from the constraints and economic pressures involved in trying to "make it" as a rock star, movie star or sports star. It allows those of us with a passion for music, acting or sports to embrace the activity for its inherent pleasures and rewards. Many of the people I interviewed, such as Michael Simkins, seem to have embraced this approach from the start, or at least came to it at some point in their career. My friend and SXSW tour guide, CJ Murdoch, is fully aware that he will never make buckets of money or achieve fame in the world of music. Despite this, he made the exact opposite decision that Rachel made. He turned his back on a successful legal career to live the life of a working musician. "When I started down this path," CJ told me, "I took a hard look at the things I have to give up to commit to a career in an area where uncertainty is lord: owning a house, getting married, having kids. I'm prepared to not have any of those things."

CJ's picture of his austere future life is a long way from the "big bucks," "big mansion," "living the high life" celebrity aspirations disclosed in the public perception research cited at the start of this second part of the book. But why would CJ make such a commitment? As he told me while we watched one of his friends perform on a tiny, unofficial SXSW stage, "I do it because I love it. I love the lifestyle. I love being on the road. And I love making music." In other words, it makes him happy.

When I returned home from my trip to New York my kids were intrigued by my discussions with struggling actors and musicians. The Caulfield family loves pop culture. I told them about Ramesh and the breakthrough audition that led to his winning a spot on *Law and Order*. When the date of the Ramesh episode arrived I watched with my cop-show-loving daughter, Alison. About forty-five minutes into the show, during a scene in a hospital, Ramesh appeared on-screen, for about ten seconds. He opened a door, approached a woman in a hospital bed, handed her a paper and said his one line, "You've been served!"

PART III

THE ILLUSION THAT CELEBRITY STATUS IS WORTH HAVING

CHAPTER 11

A LONELY, HEALTH-DESTROYING GRIND?

So, we have seen that obtaining a celebrity job is so rare that it borders on the impossible. Nevertheless, nabbing one is widely perceived as a reasonable, and obtainable, goal. Indeed, pursuing rock star, sports star or movie star fame seems often to be cast as a noble pursuit ("reach for the stars!"), albeit one that can consume a significant amount of time and financial resources. This raises another interesting question: why would anyone want to be a celebrity? Sure, the entertainment industry has many individuals working in it who are happy and fulfilled, just as any sector of society does. But if you believe the research and, for that matter, many of the featured stories in the celebrity media, being a bona fide celebrity seems to be about as rewarding as a prison sentence. And there is a bit of research to back this proposition.

Studies consistently show that being in a solid relationship is good for you. Research tells us it benefits our mental health and stress levels and is linked to living a long life. A 2006 paper in the *Journal of Health and Social Behavior* went so far as to suggest that "the evidence linking social relationships to health and mortality is as strong as that linking cigarette smoking, blood pressure, and obesity to health." A 2010 review of the evidence, published in *PLoS Medicine* came to a similar conclusion, suggesting that the "influence of social relationships on the risk of death are comparable with well-established risk factors for mortality such as smoking and alcohol consumption and exceed the influence of other risk factors such as physical inactivity and obesity." Other studies have consistently shown that marriage, in particular, is good for health. And this is especially true for us men (likely because we can barely take care of ourselves). Evidence from large cohort studies—big studies that follow large groups of individuals over a long period—have found that married men have a 46 percent lower rate of premature death than unmarried men.

So, in terms of well-being and health, relationships, particularly with a "significant other," matter. They matter a lot. But, as everyone on planet Earth (and every assiduous reader of *People* magazine) likely knows, being a celebrity is tough on relationships. The divorce rate among celebrities is much higher than the already grim divorce stats for the general public, which hover around 40 to 50 percent. Some estimates put the divorce rate for professional athletes somewhere between 60 and 80 percent. And I have had bouts of the stomach flu that have lasted longer than some celebrity marriages. (Britney Spears and Jason Allen Alexander were married for just fifty-five hours.) In fact, celebrity divorces are so predictable that they are, um, entirely predictable.

In 2006, *New York Times* columnist and social psychologist John Tierny and science writer Garth Sundem came up with a formula for forecasting the duration of celebrity marriages. It considers variables such as age, the relative fame of the husband and wife, their marital history (i.e., how many divorces are already on the books) and the degree to which they are regarded as sex symbols. This formula successfully predicted the breakup of Demi Moore and Ashton Kutcher, Pamela Anderson and Kid Rock, and Britney Spears and Kevin Federline, among others. As succinctly summarized by Tierny in a follow-up article published in 2012, "Fame, as measured by Google hits, is no good for a marriage."

Of course, celebrity brings with it many hazards, including the not insignificant fact that it might cause you to die before your time. A much-publicized 2012 study, "Dying to be Famous," compared the mortality of 1,489 rock and pop stars to that of the general, non-famous public. While the relationship between fame and mortality varied depending on the characteristics of performers—solo careers appear to be particularly risky—the study found that, in general, "mortality increases relative to the general population with time since fame." A similar 2007 study looked into the life expectancy of more than one thousand musicians involved in the top one thousand all-time albums, and noted, "From 3 to 25 years post fame, both North American and European pop stars experience significantly higher mortality (more than 1.7 times) than demographically matched populations in the USA and UK, respectively." Yet another study, published in 2013, looked at mortality across all the fame-oriented professions, including acting, sports, music, singing and dance. The authors, who examined one thousand obituaries in *The New York Times*, found that individuals in celebrity-oriented professions died at a younger age. They concluded, "Fame and achievement in performance-related careers may be earned at the cost of a shorter life expectancy."

To be fair, few studies have been published on the other side of the health-risks-of-celebrity debate. Some research suggests that a higher social rank causes animals, including humans, to live longer. Similarly, a 2008 study found that winning a Nobel Prize increases the longevity of a winner, at least over an individual who was merely nominated, by one to two years. Some speculate that the status from the award gives winners a degree of psychological resiliency that allows them to handle stress better and, as a result, they live longer. However, a much more modest "social rank" effect was found in other research that focused more closely on the world of actual celebrities. (I doubt most Nobel winners experience the same substance abuse, relationship instability and privacy pressures encountered by, say, Justin Bieber.) A 2011 study of actors who win an Academy Award found little evidence to suggest that the status they gained conferred significant life-extending benefits.

In total, while it is tough to do quality research on the issue and there are only a few less-than-methodologically-ideal studies on point, it seems fair to conclude that fame isn't all that good for your health. The increased mortality is likely due to a combination of factors, including the lack of solid relationships and the embrace of risky and health-destroying behaviors (smoking, drinking, drugs, crazy diets). However, some have speculated that the stress associated with the pressure to achieve and sustain celebrity status could also be a contributing factor. Richard Epstein, an oncologist and co-author of the obituary study noted above, has pointed to the destructive effect of the psychological and family pressures that favor high public achievement. In an interview for the Australian Broadcasting Corporation, Epstein was asked if the take-home message from this research was *Don't aspire to be famous*. His response: "I think that's what I'd tell my children.

I think I'd be very worried if my children were too fixated on achieving stardom."

Still, the rich and famous are, at least, famous and rich. Their lives may be slightly shorter, but at least they have lots of money, right? In fact, things look pretty depressing in this domain too. Even if you are lucky enough to make buckets of money through some celebrity-oriented profession, history tells us that the wealth may not last. So many high-profile celebrities have declared bankruptcy that it almost seems the norm. Consider this list of stars who have gone broke: MC Hammer, Larry King, Burt Reynolds, Willie Nelson, Mike Tyson, child actor (and once the highest paid on TV) Gary Coleman, singer Toni Braxton (twice!), Grammy winner Lauryn Hill, and football great and ten-time Pro Bowler Lawrence Taylor. Celebrity bankruptcies are so common that they may have altered the public's attitude toward bankruptcy. Business professor Rafael Efrat has argued that by publicizing celebrities' bankruptcy filings, "the media may have shaped public perception on the subject making the traditional bankruptcy stigma less pronounced."

Just how often do celebrities get into financial trouble? While I could find no scientific examination of the percentage of celebrities who go broke, a bit of data available from the sports world gives a sense of how infrequent financial stability can be for the famous. A 2009 *Sports Illustrated* investigation into the finances of professional athletes reported that 78 percent of former NFL players have "gone bankrupt or are under financial stress because of joblessness or divorce" and "within five years of retirement, an estimated 60 percent of former NBA players are broke." Since the length of a professional athlete's career is extremely short—in the NFL, for example, the average is somewhere between 3.5 and 6 years, depending on how you count—these are likely young men, many without marketable skills beyond their athletic abilities. (And remember how vanishingly rare it is to become successful enough in any celebrity profession to make money that you can then lose.)

So maybe being a celebrity is not all it's cracked up to be. In fact, few actual studies have been performed to test this proposition. One of those, published in 2009, involved in-depth and prolonged interviews with fifteen high-profile celebrities, including individuals from the worlds of acting, music and sports. The authors' goal was to get a sense of what it is like to be famous. What are the advantages and disadvantages? The celebrities were not named, but I can report, after chatting with one of the authors, that they were authentically successful and well known. Naturally, they listed the expected benefits, such as material wealth (which, as noted, is not always sustained), privileged access (again, temporary, unless celebrity status continues) and a feeling of symbolic immortality. But the interviewees also disclosed many significant downsides, including loss of privacy, feelings of isolation, the inability to trust others and the need to create a "character split" between the celebrity entity and the private self. This split can cause significant personal challenges. As Elvis Presley observed, "The image is one thing and the human being is another. It's very hard to live up to an image, put it that way." The celebrities complained about the need to always "be on," that "you are an animal in a cage" and that "being a famous person is a full-time job" (something I also heard numerous times while I was doing this research). In total, you certainly don't get the sense that these celebrities were exceptionally happy or felt as though they lived in Shangri-la or had found the pot of gold at the end of the rainbow. On the contrary, the authors note that many report a "sense of loneliness at the center of the fanfare of fame."

"This remains one of the only studies on how celebrities truly feel about being famous. But given how important the concept of celebrity is to our society, we need more work on the topic," Donna Rockwell, the lead author, tells me. Rockwell is a clinical psychologist. Prior to doing her PhD she worked in the celebrity universe as a TV journalist and producer, and it was this background that gave her access to the celebrities she interviewed. I tell her that my general impression is that a sadness permeates what she heard from celebrities. "Yes, there is an unrelenting darkness there," Rockwell says. "The isolation, the lack of trust and the loss of privacy wears on them ... celebrity life often leaves them feeling empty and broken."

These issues are bad enough for those who are currently at the peak of their celebrity, but for those whose fame-enhanced status has lost its luster, the psychological issues can be even worse. It is no fun being a former celebrity. For the no-longer-famous, it's often all downside (loss of privacy, isolation) and no upside (money, privileged access). Many former stars spend the rest of their lives being asked, "Didn't you used to be ... ?" The implication, of course, is that they aren't "someone" now. One of the subjects in her study is a singer who was the lead in one of the "greatest singing groups of her time," as Rockwell reports in her article. While her name is still known around the globe, she is now broke and struggles from day to day. "It is really heart-breaking," Rockwell says.

Rockwell cautions that we need to be careful not to generalize the results of her study too broadly; she interviewed only fifteen subjects, after all. Undoubtedly some celebrities feel happy, fulfilled, rich and, well, on-top-of-the-world fabulous. Still, her work provides valuable insight into the harsh realities that can accompany celebrity life. It also raises interesting questions about why so many people want to be a celebrity. "Anyone who has fame and celebrity as a goal needs to see a psychiatrist," Rockwell says only half jokingly. "It really makes no rational sense."

THE LITTLE HOUSE OF HEDONIC ADAPTATION

All the women in my house love *Little House on the Prairie*. They love the books, the TV show and the entire Little House gestalt. My eldest daughter has dressed up as the main character, Laura Ingalls, for Halloween. Twice. So has my wife, Joanne. My poor parenting skills are often compared to the unflappable, ever-capable and deeply caring approach of *Little House* patriarch Charles "Pa" Ingalls—as in, "I don't think Pa would have handled it [fight / upset child / milking of a cow] that way" or "Pa could probably fix it [plugged toilet / leaky roof / broken promise due to airing of important NFL game]." And power outages are viewed as a terrific opportunity to live life "Ingalls style."

As a result, my status on the home front rose considerably when I announced that I would be interviewing Alison Arngrim, the actor who played Laura Ingalls's nemesis, the spoiled and conniving Nellie Oleson. The character of Nellie, with her curly blond hair (a very expensive wig, it turns out) and stuck-up nose, was a central part of the *Little House* narrative. As a general rule, everyone who loves the show despises Nellie. To do otherwise would be akin to cheering for Snidely Whiplash to defeat Dudley Do-Right or for Darth Vader to lure Luke to the dark side. Indeed, as revealed in Arngrim's wonderful 2010 autobiography, her very first acting review had more than a dash of venom. Arngrim was twelve. The review was delivered in a loud, clear voice by a classmate hanging out a second-story window during a school recess break: *"You biiiiitchhh!!!"* "There are many who still think of me that way," Arngrim tells me. "People approach me in restaurants to let me know! Some of it is tongue in cheek, some of it is not."

For those too young to remember the show, some history and context is likely in order. *Little House on the Prairie,* which aired from 1974 to 1983, followed the life of a nineteenth-century American farm family. It was tremendously popular. The Nellie Oleson character was so cruel to the sweet and always-kind Laura Ingalls that she quickly became an icon of evil, so much so that *Vanity Fair* once declared Nellie Oleson to be the number-one female villain in TV history. Syndication of the show—it has run in more than 140 countries—has allowed the Nellie aversion to live on. *Little House* is *still* shown on numerous channels throughout the world.

Arngrim meets me in a well-known bar in the heart of West Hollywood. As we chat, a few patrons stop by to say they are fans. Just as Arngrim starts telling me about the enduring loathing people harbor for Nellie, a woman, as if on cue, points at Arngrim and says, "I used to hate you." Arngrim smiles, waves and says thanks. No edge or bitterness. She comes across as friendly, warm and genuine—one of those immediately likable people. This is Nellie Oleson? Nope.

"Why would anyone want to be famous? It is not that much fun," Arngrim tells me. And she should know. Not only did *Little*

House make her very famous, she grew up in the midst of famous people. Her parents were involved in the entertainment business and her brother was also a successful child actor. At one point her family lived in the Chateau Marmont, a Hollywood hotel with a celebrity-rich history that includes famous deaths (John Belushi died of a drug overdose in a hotel bungalow), injuries (Jim Morrison, who briefly lived in the hotel, fell off a balcony), romantic encounters (Clark Gable and Jean Harlow) and, of course, epic parties. For a good part of her life, she literally lived in a celebrity-filled world. It was her norm.

But Arngrim also spent many years struggling with the costs of fame, the challenge of trying to transition into an adult star (this included roles on shows like *The Love Boat* and *Fantasy Island* that were calculated to be provocative), and then life as a "former" star. She has an intimate knowledge of both the celebrity world and the impact of the various shades of fame on one's life.

So, why *do* people want to be famous? As noted in previous chapters, there are many possible explanations, including a range of hardwired cognitive biases and the peculiar pressure exerted by popular culture. But what are people *seeking* in celebrity life? And why don't the harsh realities of celebrity existence dissuade more? My review of the research exploring this issue highlights several relatively obvious themes, including a desire for wealth, a luxurious lifestyle, attention, admiration and status, and the sense that celebrity will grant a degree of symbolic immortality. In his book *Look at Me: The Fame Motive from Childhood to*

Death, Orville Gilbert Brim speculated that the desire for fame flows from the basic human need for acceptance and approval, and that it is intensified in some children due to less-than-ideal early-life relationships. It is, in other words, a built-in desire that, for some, is intensified by life circumstances. "The fame motive will not go away but must be endured as a kind of chronic hunger," Brim writes, "never completely satisfied for the rest of one's life."

While Brim's depiction may seem a bit grim and hyperbolic (a chronic hunger?), some recent empirical work supports his view. A study published in 2013 used an online survey to explore the personality tendencies that are associated with the appeal of fame. The authors found that higher "belongingness needs"— that is, a strong desire to feel accepted and included—were associated with an increased interest in all aspects of fame (e.g., having status, being well known and highly visible, and having the support of family and friends). It isn't necessary for me to go into too much detail about the psychological traits of individuals who have a strong or near pathological desire for fame (though I will talk about narcissism below); readers will agree, I think, that it is a social trend that is gaining strength. That said, research suggests that the desire for fame is associated with a number of identifiable personality characteristics, including a particular vulnerability and desire to make one's life better. A 2010 study by John Maltby, for example, found, among other relevant personality traits, "an interest in fame emerging as a desire to overcome negative feelings about oneself and their well-being and happiness" and a lack of confidence that leads to a desire "to escape aspects of their current life or character by becoming famous." John Gountas at Murdoch University surveyed more than five hundred individuals for a study published in 2012. A clear materialistic theme emerged: simply put, some people want to be famous to get the tangible benefits of fame. Celebrity status, he reported, is seen as "a vehicle for the achievement of a particular lifestyle that satisfies personal goals." Gountas subsequently commented that he was motivated to do the work because he believes the increasing desire for fame is "not just a blip on our radar, but actually a large social and cultural change among young people."

It seems to me that these findings go to the heart of the illusion that achieving fame and celebrity will confer certain benefits and will, ultimately, make us happy, which, we now know, is far from a certain outcome. As Marilyn Monroe once said, "Fame doesn't fulfill you. It warms you a bit, but that warmth is temporary."

Like Monroe, Arngrim does not see fame or celebrity as an avenue to happiness or self-improvement. On the contrary, "Being famous is hard," she says after reflecting on the struggles of Justin Bieber, Cory Monteith, Mischa Barton, Paris Jackson and other young celebrities. "It should never be the goal. If you are unhappy, getting famous is the biggest mistake. Fame doesn't fix problems, it amplifies them. Gasoline on a flame. A small problem becomes a gigantic one." To support this bleak assessment, Arngrim points to the numerous celebrity suicides and suicide attempts. I could find no definitive scientific data to back up her speculation, but some media reports have suggested that celebrities, particularly those who have acquired fame via reality TV, commit suicide at a higher rate than the general public. While there is, obviously, a causation issue (is it celebrity life that is the problem or does the prospect of celebrity attract individuals who are more likely to be psychologically fragile?), we can say with a degree of certainty, I think, that little evidence, anecdotal or otherwise, supports the notion that fame will help to resolve psychological issues.

One study, published in 2013, examined the circumstances attending the suicide of seventy-two celebrities. Using biographies as source material, the authors found that in 97 percent of the cases, a tension existed between the individual's aspiration for success and the reality of his or her situation. In other words, at the time of their death, the celebrities wanted to be more successful than they were. The authors hypothesize that this strain may contribute to the risk of suicide. They also note that celebrities are, in general, unusually ambitious, and consequently it should be no surprise that their aspirations outstrip objective assessments of their chance of success—a point we have touched on throughout this book.

Suicide is a tremendously complex phenomenon with causations that are, as a psychiatrist colleague observed, idiosyncratic and personal. We should take care not to over-interpret the conclusions from this study. Still, the research raises intriguing questions about the psychological impact of our society's love affair with a celebrity-oriented, reach-for-the-stars kind of ambition, especially given the illusory nature of both the goal and the chance of success.

At this point, you might be thinking that all this negativity sounds like sour grapes. I failed at my lame attempts at rock 'n' roll glory, so now I am trying to rationalize my mundane existence. This is a logical—and probably not entirely inaccurate—assessment. Also, as noted, some celebrities are perfectly content. So, in order to provide a bit of balance, it is fair to consider the genuine advantages of fame. With this in mind, I searched the popular press for any celebrity quote that described the perks of fame. This approach, I admit, was far from methodologically rigorous. The celebrities could be lying, the quote could be from a publicist and many of the comments come from sources such as *People* magazine, which is hardly a repository of deep thinking. Still, I did find a pretty consistent, and oddly food-oriented, theme.

Most celebrities admit that they love the special treatment and day-to-day conveniences afforded by fame. Who wouldn't? As Woody Allen said recently, "You get better seats at the basketball game, and you get better tables and reservations [at] places, and if I call a doctor on Saturday morning I can get him." Actor Chris O'Donnell (*Batman and Robin*, *Scent of a Woman* and *NCIS: Los Angeles*) said, "The best thing about being famous is getting a nice table at a restaurant." Kelly Clarkson also likes having the ability to drop her name to get a restaurant reservation. Apparently she has an assistant do the name-dropping. "I've never dropped it myself though, I'd feel like a tool." (Yes, Kelly, having your personal assistant drop your name is much less tool-ish than doing it yourself.) Jennifer Lawrence, who has said that fame has ruined her personal life, likes the little things, such as being able to take stuff from the minibar in her hotel room. Actor Jessica Chastain (*Zero Dark Thirty* and *The Help*) appreciates the access to and opportunity to wear designer clothes. Britney Spears says, "The cool thing about being famous is traveling. I have always wanted to travel across seas, like to Canada and stuff." (Real quote. Not the best example, admittedly, but I just couldn't resist.)

Even *Twilight* star Robert Pattinson, who has had few good things to say about fame, admits he likes "staying in fancy hotels with incredibly nice bathrooms."

Another big draw and, I suppose, a genuine benefit to the celebrity life is the unique social access it facilitates. In her book *Starstruck: The Business of Celebrity*, Elizabeth Currid-Halkett suggests that being a celebrity is like belonging to a members-only club. "They are a part of a very elite invite-only network," Currid-Halkett writes. Indeed, this celebrity club is a real and measurable phenomenon. Currid-Halkett's analysis of celebrity networks found that celebrities "exhibit just 3.26 degrees of separation from one another," far less than the well-known "six degrees of separation." They hang together, know each other and gravitate to the same social gatherings. Wanting entrance to this "club," and the perceived (and highly publicized) advantages it provides—private parties, movie premieres, award shows and career-enhancing friendships—is an understandable goal.

But, as we have seen, all this glamour and excitement will not, necessarily, make a person feel happier or more fulfilled. Nor will money. Research has consistently shown that after hitting middle-class levels of income, or slightly higher, further increases in wealth do little to heighten happiness. Indeed, because of a process called hedonic adaptation, the thrill that these experiences and advantages provide quickly fades. As Fyodor Dostoyevsky astutely observed, "Man is a pliant animal, a being who gets accustomed to anything." This includes, I am sure Fyodor would agree, getting a good table at a restaurant.

This phenomenon is supported by numerous empirical studies. One of the most famous, published in 1978, compared the happiness of twenty-two major lottery winners with that of twenty-nine paralyzed accident victims. Amazingly, the lottery winners were *not* happier and, in fact, they took less pleasure in the ordinary aspects of life. While subsequent research has tweaked these results, the general premise—that people tend to revert to a kind of "happiness baseline" regardless of circumstances—has been experimentally replicated many times. This process may be an evolutionary adaptation that causes the stimuli we face in our day-to-day lives, whether it is an awesome Paleolithic cave, an attractive spouse or a new Lamborghini, to fade into the background. This allows us to concentrate on novel stimuli, which are usually, from a survival point of view, the better use of our mental resources. Also, if we did not adapt to new circumstances, we would not continue to strive for new achievements, a compulsion that may also have evolutionary benefits. This adaptation happens regardless of the positive (marriage, a birth) or negative (divorce, a death in the family) nature of the event. Our subjective well-being requires us to adapt to whatever the circumstances are. While people often do not fully rebound from all negative events (unemployment, the onset of a disability), we are generally remarkably resilient. And people seem to adapt more consistently and completely to positive events. No matter how big the achievement, perk or reward, the boost in happiness doesn't last long and our level of happiness returns to the baseline. So, while getting a great table at a restaurant, traveling first class, hanging with other celebs, and going to movie premieres is exciting at first, we get used to it. The buzz diminishes. Then, remarkably quickly, the perks don't seem like perks and they do little to boost happiness.

Katherine Bao studies happiness at Manhattanville College. She tells me that "people adapt pretty quickly to material purchases," so it seems unlikely that celebrity privileges will result in any kind of continued happiness. "Having the latest gadgets and shiny new cars will only make a person happy for so long," she says. And there's also the matter of social comparison. Because celebrities often inhabit a celebrity network, their perks don't seem so special. "Such upward social comparison could mean that their purchases bring them even less happiness than they would someone who is not so aware of what others have or who is surrounded by people who have less than them."

Ambition is another highly relevant reason people rapidly adapt to positive events. As soon as a goal is achieved—landing a new job, getting a part in a movie—people have a tendency to look for the next rung on the ladder leading to success and happiness. Research has found that having lofty aspirations is a predictor of *lower* well-being, especially if those aspirations relate to extrinsic goals (money, fame, rewards) as compared to intrinsic goals (self-acceptance, community feeling). Bao cautioned that the relationship between aspirations and happiness is complex. For example, people with high aspirations are often happy, but "at some point aspirations may become so high that they are essentially impossible to achieve, and our research shows that when people fail to fulfill their aspirations, their happiness declines."

Another study, published in 2012, involving some five hundred students, revealed that constantly aspiring for *more* happiness equated with decreased happiness in the present. The authors, psychologists Kennon Sheldon and Sonja Lyubomirsky, concluded that "striving for ever-greater happiness may set one on a hedonic treadmill to nowhere." Once again, the observation seems particularly relevant to our reach-for-the-stars society and to those pursuing the essentially unattainable goal of celebrity—stuck on a treadmill to nowhere.

The disadvantages to being a celebrity are generally well known. They are the stuff of headlines and celebrity biographies. They serve as fodder for entertainment journalists and gossip columnists. Much of Perez Hilton's online success, for instance, is built on mapping the misfortunes of celebrities. So it is worth considering why the negatives do not, in the eyes of aspiring celebrities, overwhelm the positives. Why don't people worry about all the bad stuff associated with fame? The biggest reason, I suspect, is one we have already covered: optimistic bias. People simply do not think that bad things are going to happen to them. And they see their future in an overly optimistic light: they believe their chance of achieving a desired goal is better than average and are terrible at guessing what it will be like when they achieve it. "When *I* become a celebrity," the thinking goes, "I will get all the benefits and none of the bad stuff. I won't blow my money. I will appreciate my good fortune. I will be able to handle fame. I will stay in a good relationship. I will not have addiction problems. Etc., etc."

Daniel Gilbert, a psychologist at Harvard University, has spent decades studying and writing about why individuals make particular life choices and how those choices get screwed up. He has demonstrated that, sure enough, people overestimate their chance of success. In general, our view of what life will be like once our goals are achieved is overwhelmingly positive and largely inaccurate. "Few people see the negative consequences of being a celebrity. They fail to imagine all the complications of celebrity life," Gilbert tells me. "They don't think about the day-to-day reality. How they live their lives." In part, this is because we are constantly bombarded by unrealistic representations of celebrity existence. Pictures of celebrity homes, fashion, parties and cars are absolutely everywhere. This plays into a number of our cognitive biases. For example, as Gilbert has noted in his research, if something is easy to imagine—say, a fabulous lifestyle—you may think it is more likely to happen than a more objective assessment would dictate. This tendency is tied to several cognitive biases, including confirmation bias (the tendency to give more weight and attention to data that support a belief) and the availability heuristic (the ease to which we can bring something to mind), among others.

I decide to test my theory that a constant bombardment of positive representations of celebrity life feeds our cognitive biases. I walk into a bookstore and go to the entertainment section of the magazine stand. My goal is to pick up every magazine that covers celebrities and see if they have at least one story, such as a feature on a spectacular house, vacation home or apartment, that highlights the fabulous celebrity lifestyle. To document my work, I intend to take a picture of both the cover of the magazine and the relevant story. I confess that the thoroughness of my investigation is seriously hampered by the embarrassing nature of my task.

"Excuse me, can I help you?" a young female clerk asks me as I start collecting my "data." Picture how this must look to her. I am a middle-aged man awkwardly taking camera-phone pictures of starlets, some in bikinis, on the cover of gossip magazines. "I am, um, doing research … kind of," I reply. She clearly does not believe me, but slowly walks away. She gives me one last over-the-shoulder glare. I forge ahead, but only get through nine magazines before shame overwhelms me. Here are the results of my clumsy investigation:

Hello! Magazine: "Kim Wilde [a UK pop star/presenter/ model]: Inviting Us into Her Stunning 16th Century Retreat."

US Weekly: A bikini-clad Kim Kardashian is on the cover (I can't escape this woman). She is "slamming the fat bullies" for their mean comments about her pregnancy physique and declaring, "My Body Is Back, No Gimmicks, No Surgery." It is portrayed as a triumph. Revenge. A quick flip through the magazine reveals no stories that are explicitly about celebrity domiciles, but there is one on Jennifer Aniston's most recent holiday bash. That's close enough.

Life and Style Weekly: This has an article on the "Fabulous Life of Blake Lively." It includes a detailed description of her $2.35 million "Cosy Country Retreat," to which she is "putting personal touches" because "Martha Stewart is her idol."

People: As a regular reader, I have seen dozens of stories about celebrity homes. It is almost a regular feature. Indeed, by my rough calculations, more than 80 percent of the issues have at least one story about a cool celebrity home, vacation, etc. In the issue I hold in the bookstore, the best example is a story entitled "The Jolie-Pitts Australian Adventures," about how the "most glamorous party of eight" spends its time Down Under. (As I write this, People.com also has an online quiz entitled "Insane

Celebrity Homes!: From multimillion-dollar estates to homes with moats (seriously!)." It encourages us to take the test to find out "how well you know the domiciles of the rich and famous!" I clearly don't. Despite more than a year of immersion in celebrity culture, I get every question wrong.)

In Touch: This magazine, like so many others in this genre, takes a yin/yang approach to celebrity life. The cover has a headline that reads "I'm Lucky to Be Alive: Drugs, Arrests, Psych Wards ..." The story is about the troubled life of former child star Amanda Bynes. But things get much more cheery later with a feature called "Crib of the Week." It is a story about actor couple Diane Kruger (*Troy*, *Inglourious Basterds*) and Joshua Jackson (*Fringe*, *Dawson's Creek*) selling their Hollywood "Hillside Hideway," despite having fabulous neighbors such as Drew Barrymore, Zac Efron and Katy Perry.

Star: This publication has a piece on Ricky Martin's $8.3-million high-rise pad in Manhattan, which, I am sure, affords Ricky many opportunities to live *la vida loca*.

Closer Weekly: I have never heard of this periodical. The catch-phrase above the title says its goal is to bring me closer to the stars I love. As a result of this unabashed embrace of a voyeuristic ethos, the magazine naturally has much on celebrity lifestyles, including a six-page spread on Jeff Probst's home or, as he calls it, "the house that *Survivor* built."

Scandalous: This big, glossy magazine looks like a one-off publication focused on the reckless lifestyles of the rich and famous (so, basically, a magazine about divorce, breakdowns, drugs, bankruptcy and arrests). But I am including it in this list because it has an article entitled "Rehab Retreats for the Rich and Famous." One of these facilities, the magazine claims, costs $60,000 a month.

Of course, this is a survey of just one magazine stand and of the stories that cover just the amazing places where celebrities live. I could have undertaken a similar survey focused on clothes. There is almost always a "best-dressed" section in these magazines. Another big theme: celebrity kids. It seems as if every edition of *People* magazine has a two-page photo spread showing celebrities hanging with their adorable children. Or I could have looked at TV shows or Twitter feeds from sources like TMZ or E! Online.

It is no surprise, Gilbert explains, that people would be enticed by these representations. "There is no reason to believe that social comparison theory doesn't apply to [individuals looking up to] celebrities," he observes. In other words, we upward compare to the fantasy world created by lifestyle reporting. Compared to the celebrity homes portrayed in entertainment magazines, most of us live in relative deprivation. And, as with beauty and body image, social media both intensifies and increases the availability of images that play into our cognitive biases. Formats such as Facebook and Twitter "bring us closer to celebrities," Gilbert says. Recent studies consistently show the power of new media to increase the sway of celebrity culture, for good and bad. Authors of a study published in 2013 interviewed forty-five of Lady Gaga's fans (as of writing, she has 41 million Twitter followers). They found that new media, particularly Twitter, created an illusion that individuals were interacting directly with the star. While such interactions can be beneficial, providing support for individuals who feel isolated, we should not underestimate the power of social media forums to serve as a vehicle for social comparison. "They are a stage for bragging. 'Look what I've got!'" Gilbert says. "This makes us feel bad. Most aspirations are set by looking around and seeing what others have."

And, if you believe what you see in social media and the entertainment media, celebrities have a lot!

The quest for fame often starts in our teen years and this ties into another reason why the downsides of celebrity life have little effect on our society's endemic quest for fame. Teenagers are notoriously oblivious to risk—particularly if the risk is likely to manifest in the far future. As biological entities, teenagers are pretty here-and-now focused. As philosopher Adam Smith famously noted, "The contempt of risk and the presumptuous hope of success are in no period of life more active than at the age at which young people choose their professions."

A large body of research has backed up Smith's eighteenth-century speculation. Some studies, for example, suggest that the teenage brain is wired to take on risks or, at least, perceive them differently than the adult brain. It is no surprise, then, that teenagers are willing to do some pretty crazy and dangerous things to achieve celebrity status. According to one study, for instance, 57 percent of people already taking steroids would take a pill or supplement in order to achieve future sports success even if they were sure it would shorten their life. There is little evidence that the well-publicized risks associated with concussions in football and hockey have dissuaded any rising stars from playing. And UK teachers told researchers that becoming a celebrity is often a primary goal for their teenage students. Indeed, many of their students are willing to quit school to achieve it—which, I would suggest, is a fairly high-risk career strategy.

I can relate to this kind of risk taking. I was certain I was going to make it in the music industry. That certainty crystallized in my late teens. My mom—who provided advice in a very hands-off manner, parenting mostly by stealth—was supportive of my music aspirations, but constantly pushed education. "Do whatever makes you happy," she would say, "but promise me you will get a university education." I came close to breaking that promise on several occasions. The pressure to hit the road with a struggling band emerged almost every year while I pursued my undergraduate degree. Sometimes I wonder what would have happened if I didn't hate being in a moving vehicle as much as I do. Did my fear of motion sickness keep me in school?

Back in West Hollywood, Arngrim muses on the attraction fame has for children and adolescents. "When you are a kid it is normal to dream," Arngrim says. "But grown-ups are supposed to know it is nuts." The combination of adolescent risk taking and a deep parental belief that is skewed by various cognitive biases has likely propelled many an individual toward the search for celebrity status.

Paul Petersen could not agree more with Arngrim. "Why would parents wish this on their kids? Human beings have blinders on." Like Arngrim, Petersen knows Hollywood and what it is like to be famous. He started his acting career on the *Mickey*

Mouse Club when he was just ten. He was in a movie with Cary Grant and Sophia Loren and was on the popular *Donna Reed Show* from 1958 to 1966. More important for my purposes, he is the founder of an organization called A Minor Consideration. The goal of this foundation is to provide guidance and support for young performers. (Visitors to its website will find, among other sensible recommendations, that "child stars must pick their parents with care.") As the foundation's head, Petersen has had the opportunity to work closely with many young celebrities, past and present. He also aims to educate parents about the business ("it is show *business*, not show *fun*"); about the reality of making it (very few can sustain a long career because, he says, "you *will* fall out of fashion"); and all the lifestyle risks. He wants parents and children to know that "when you sacrifice the developmental years of your life, you will pay the price." But despite his best efforts, his message often does not get through. "Parents always think they can do it ... beat the odds. Parents think the bad things won't happen. They ignore the advice."

FORM LETTER TO NUTTY PARENTS

Dear "Committed" Parent at My Kid's Hockey/Dance/Music/etc. Class:

Re: The Nurturing of Your Kid's "Special" Talents

I realize that you want the best for your kid. I realize that you believe he/she is uniquely talented. My kids are super-amazing too (except most of the time). But I am not sure you have thought through your plans for world domination in [hockey/dance/

singing/etc.]. Let's do the math. (1) The chance of making it big is approximately zero. Do not let confirmation bias fool you. Your kid is not going to be a world-renowned star. It is not going to happen. (2) And even if it does happen (and I can't emphasize this enough, it probably won't), there is a good chance that he/she will be divorced, broke and unemployed before he/she hits the age of thirty. [Note: If the kid is in hockey, add "head-injured," and if in popular music, add "struggling with addiction."] Also, perhaps most importantly, research tells us there is a good chance he/she will not be happy. You are, in effect, wishing for your kid a life of financial misery, isolation and lost opportunities. Is this a good idea?

I fully appreciate that I am coming off like a patronizing know-it-all jerk and that you will likely feel compelled to punch me in the face the next time you see me. Please don't. I have a delicate jaw. And besides, this letter was actually [neighbor's name]'s idea.

Yours truly,

[If brave, your name here. If not, insert spouse's name.]

p.s., I understand from [neighbor's name] that you were a pretty good [hockey player/dancer/singer/etc.]. Sorry that didn't work out for you.

Individuals often strive for celebrity status because their parents have nudged them in that direction. And, no surprise, this often happens because parents want to live vicariously through their kids. A study published in 2013 provides the first empirical data on the idea that parents use their children to fulfill their own broken dreams. "Parents may come to see their children as symbols for their own success," the authors write, "and desire them to fulfill the ambitions they once held for themselves." It was a relatively small experiment—involving just seventy-three parents—for such a complex topic. Its authors focused on what the parents had to say about their ambitions for their children, rather than tracking actual parental behaviors. Nevertheless, the study provides empirical support for the notion that parents see their children as extensions of themselves, and transfer to their children their own failed attempts at glory.

Most of us will recognize this phenomenon from our own experience. Many of us have seen it play out in hockey rinks, where we encounter little kids with $300 hockey sticks; at dance studios, where stage mothers primp two-year-olds; and at music recitals, where parents encourage their prodigies to spend more time practicing than sleeping. Other studies have found that people regret lost opportunities more than anything else. Nothing burns like the memory of an unfulfilled dream. So, the compulsion to make up for lost opportunities through our children is hardly surprising.

And that reminds me, why the heck won't any of my kids start a rock band? They'd be great!

Three hours after we started our discussion, Arngrim is still laughing, smiling and willing to chat. The woman has a million stories. All good. I am sure Nellie would not have been so generous with her time or half as fun to hang out with. She tells me she is now happy. Her life is a satisfying mix of performing, writing, stand-up comedy (a routine built around her persona as a "prairie bitch") and work as an AIDS activist. She has learned to embrace her Nellie past. She can't run from it, as I saw during our afternoon together, so she has found a constructive place for Nellie to hang. Perhaps not right on her shoulder, but never far from view.

Before we part, I want to ask her one last question. As we have seen, the combination of social pressure to "reach for the stars" and a host of built-in cognitive biases creates an environment that has made celebrity seem both worthwhile and attainable. But everything is an illusion, from the chance of making it to what it will be like if it is achieved. In other words, much of our culture, many of our dreams and many of our life decisions flow from a foundation of promises and presumptions that are, in fact, no more real than the Wizard of Oz's magic. Given this reality, I ask Arngrim, why do people try?

"You know, it is just ridiculous. It [success] is just so very rare," Arngrim says emphatically.

"But people like to gamble, even if they don't think of it that way?" I note.

"Hey, I still buy lottery tickets, but I don't spend the rent," Arngrim says. "If people gambled with this kind of money in Vegas, everyone would say they had a gambling problem. But when people do it for fame and celebrity, for some bizarre reason our society says it is okay."

THE DREAM CRUSHER?

In this book I have explored the myriad ways celebrity culture presents an inaccurate or warped picture of the world. I have tried to show the degree to which celebrities—or, really, the messages that flow from celebrity culture—are wrong about almost everything, be it in relation to health, beauty, the goals to which we should aspire or definitions of the good life. But I have said little about the place, role and impact of celebrity culture in society more broadly—and much can be said (and many terrific scholars have had their say) on this point. Celebrity culture is, of course, more than just an interest in celebrities. It is a reflection of our collective values and a manifestation of complex interplay between social expectations and socioeconomic realities. As sociologist Karen Sternheimer wrote in *Celebrity Culture and the American Dream*, "Rather than simple superficial distractions, celebrity and fame are unique manifestations of our sense of American social mobility: they provide the illusion that material wealth is possible for anyone.... Celebrities seem to provide proof that the American Dream of going from rags to riches is real and attainable."

This is more than mere academic musing. A belief in the celebrity illusion can have a tangible impact on life choices.

A 2002 study of US college football players, to cite one more example, found that 84 percent of the African American players had an "expectation of a career in professional athletics" and 40 percent believed that sports is the best route to economic success. Keep in mind that these are individuals who were *in* university. One would hope they'd have a positive view about the role of education in their future. The researchers also found that those players who held these kinds of beliefs were also more likely to have "been placed on academic probation and suspension," among other less than ideal behaviors.

Given what we have covered in this book, findings of this nature are far from surprising, but they remain no less disheartening. Belief in celebrity success is built on a foundation of lies, illusions and empty exhortations of the present reach-for-the-stars variety. The chance of making it celebrity big in any kind of celebrity-oriented career hovers near zero. And even if an individual makes it big, the attainment of the goal is unlikely to provide the promised long-term wealth or, more importantly, the desired happiness and well-being. There is no pot at the end of the rainbow.

The misconceptions that exist in the context of health and beauty are just as insidious. The beauty standard set by celebrity culture is not only unrealistic but also increasingly disconnected from reality. It is a standard that has less and less to do with what humans actually look like. The bulk of health and beauty products and recommendations peddled by or through celebrities are either useless or harmful or both. They may also divert millions of individuals from engaging in the simple and evidence-based steps necessary in order to live in a health-promoting manner. Celebrity culture places aesthetics above health and well-being; values immediate results above the adoption of sustainable, long-term health strategies; and, perhaps worst of all, confuses science and pseudoscience, making it more difficult for us all to sift through the mountains of health, diet and beauty advice that permeates popular culture.

The good news is that there are things that can be done to improve our health and, even, our appearance. We can adopt a healthy lifestyle that embraces well-known and evidence-based practices that will have a measurable impact. And we can simply disregard the pseudoscientific spin that spews from the celebrity universe. With few exceptions, it is all bunk. Ignore the diets. Ignore the fitness routines. Ignore the health and beauty advice.

But we should also consider strategies to mitigate the adverse impact that celebrity culture might have on our ambitions, our definition of success and the way we view our current life circumstances. Simply learning to recognize and remind ourselves of the numerous cognitive biases that twist how we think about the world may help us to make more-informed life choices.

It is worth remembering, even if we don't really crave celebrity status, that celebrity culture can still have a significant impact on our life, by, for example, reinforcing a particular definition of success—the obtainment of wealth, a particular norm of beauty, etc.—that may tend to make us dissatisfied with our lot and to crave things that have little connection to happiness or health. Social comparisons, even to celebrity life, likely happen automatically. I am not arguing that we should settle for mediocrity, but, perhaps, we should occasionally critically appraise the nature of the goals for which we strive. Do they, for example, even exist?

"Jeez, Dad. You are kind of a downer," my eldest son, Adam, told me when we were talking about some of the themes in this book. "I am going to call you the dream crusher!" With all due respect to my son, I think he is entirely wrong. I am not denying that it is fun to dream. Nor am I suggesting that if you really want to be a singer, actor, model, dancer or professional athlete, you shouldn't aspire to that goal. But know the reality of the situation. And pursue the goal because you love the activity, the craft or the challenge, not because you want to be rich and famous. This is advice I heard again and again while working on this book. I heard it from an *American Idol* finalist, a TV producer, directors, a legendary publicist, academics, award-winning actors and many, many musicians. I view this advice not as dream crushing but as liberating. You aren't going to be rich and famous. Stop worrying about it.

Filmmaker and comedian Bobcat Goldthwait, whose most recent film, *God Bless America*, includes, coincidentally, a spoof of *American Idol*, provided this advice during a commencement speech he delivered for his daughter's graduation from college. "I truly believe that success is for creeps. We already reward narcissism way too much in our culture," he said. "Do what makes you happy, and be nice."

I'd like to end by reflecting on how this all fits into a bigger picture. I admit up front that only a thin strand of current data can be found to support the speculation that follows. But bear with me. I think this analysis provides an interesting context within which we can think about the possible role and impact of celebrity culture in modern society.

The countries that seem the most obsessed with celebrity culture (e.g., the United States, the United Kingdom, South Korea)—do not rank particularly well in rankings of population happiness. According to the 2013 *World Happiness Report*, a study prepared for the United Nations, the happiest countries in the world are Denmark, Norway and Switzerland. Canada ranks sixth. The United States and the United Kingdom, two countries that both produce and consume a great deal of celebrity culture, rank seventeenth and twenty-second respectively. These same celebrity-loving countries also have a terrible record when it comes to social mobility. The United Kingdom ranks last in the OECD and the United States is third last. In other words, in these countries, moving up the socioeconomic ladder is nearly impossible. If you are born into poverty, you are likely to stay in poverty. If you are a middle-class kid, chances are you will be a middle-class adult. Ditto your kids. (Incidentally, the country that has the highest degree of social mobility? Happy Denmark.)

Some commentators have gone so far as to call the American Dream a myth, a topic I discussed with Howard Steven Friedman, a well-known statistician with the United Nations and author of *Measure of a Nation*. "The idea of social mobility, of becoming rich, is core to the American mythology," Friedman says. "But, ironically, American performance in this area is consistently one of the worst of the developed nations." Friedman has observed that the statistics are very depressing for those "who subscribe to the notion that America is a meritocracy and a 'land of opportunity.'" And the data tell us social mobility is getting worse.

What is the best way to ensure improved social mobility, a societal goal we can all agree is important? Education. A 2012 study by the Pew Charitable Trust, *Pursuing the American Dream: Economic Mobility Across Generations*, found that "[a] four-year college degree promotes upward mobility from the bottom and prevents downward mobility from the middle and top." I ask Erin Currier, the project director for Pew's Economic Mobility Project and a co-author of the study, if education is the most important tool to the promotion of social mobility. "Absolutely. Research has shown this again and again," she says. "And what is often overlooked is that it leads not only to more mobility, but better jobs." Given this reality, it is worth noting that numerous studies, such as the OECD's regular Programme for International Student Assessment, have consistently found that the US and UK's education systems do not rank particularly well as compared to those of other developed nations.

What do all these data about happiness, education and social mobility have to do with celebrity culture? We live in a world where people increasingly turn to celebrity culture as a way of thinking about and striving for social mobility, whether through real-life choices or merely through fantasies about a life that could be, and as a means of improving our well-being, health and appearance. Is it a coincidence that countries that fare relatively poorly with respect to social mobility, happiness and education also embrace celebrity culture and a reach-for-the-stars mentality? Perhaps. (And I realize I am straying precariously close to an "opiate of the masses" thesis.) It seems hard to deny that a convergence of a variety of socioeconomic (e.g., poor social mobility) and technological (e.g., social media) trends and human psychological and social predispositions and biases have created the perfect conditions for celebrity culture to thrive.

I run this theory by Stephen Duncombe, a professor of media studies at NYU and author of *Dream: Re-Imagining Progressive Politics in an Age of Fantasy*. "This certainly seems plausible," he says. "Celebrity is so tied to democracy and succeeding, especially now. People like Kim Kardashian seem real. They act like us. They come from places that we come from. This isn't Grace Kelly. Celebrity culture makes social mobility look like magic." Indeed, it is often sold as magic. It is sold as a life-changing process that is now—or so the celebrity myth goes—increasingly available to all.

Joshua Gamson, a professor at the University of San Francisco College of Arts and Sciences and a well-known commentator on celebrity culture, tells me something similar. "In a society with tremendous income inequality, with many avenues [to success] effectively closed, here you have a way to fantasy—a get-rich-quick fantasy. You can understand why people want to keep the dream alive," he says. "The shortcut to mobility is very appealing."

Currier agrees with the take presented by Gamson and Duncombe: "It is possible that, given the barriers to social mobility, for some, they see celebrity as the only viable option." To support this view, Currier tells me of a 2006 study that found 38 percent of those with incomes below $25,000 think that winning the lottery represents the most practical way for them to accumulate wealth. Given this kind of thinking, which, as Currier noted, is likely a manifestation of a perceived lack of options, is it any surprise that so many perceive making it celebrity big as a viable goal? We could certainly quibble over the degree to which the rise in celebrity culture is a contributing cause or a by-product of existing social realities. But no matter how tenuous the connection or complex the direction of the relationship, it seems difficult to deny that our current fascination with celebrity has the potential to lead to more unhappiness—about our bodies, faces, careers, homes, clothes and even the appearance of our spouses. More importantly, this societal obsession does little to elevate or prioritize activities that will promote true social mobility and well-being. The power of celebrity culture to distract in a less than constructive manner happens on both the level of the individual (e.g., decisions about education paths, the way we think about and define success, the use of individual and family resources, etc.) and society (e.g., how the public engages with broader social issues).

A study published in 2007 found that those who "follow celebrity culture are the least engaged in politics and least likely to use their social networks to involve themselves in action or discussion about public-type issues." There is, of course, a causation issue with these kinds of data. (Perhaps those who aren't interested in social issues are attracted to celebrity culture?) Still, it shows that, at a minimum, celebrity culture does little to help, or, as noted by the authors, "it challenges suggestions of how popular culture might contribute to effective democracy."

On a more fundamental level, some research suggests that celebrity culture has contributed to the rise of a more narcissistic society. Few have done as much work on this point as Jean Twenge, a psychologist at San Diego State University and co-author of the 2009 book *The Narcissism Epidemic*. To quote from a 2013 paper by Twenge, "the overwhelming majority of the evidence shows that more recent generations of young people have more positive self-views, endorse more narcissistic personality traits, and are more self-focused." This attitude is the result of a number of factors, including our society's embrace of a reach-for-the-stars mentality and, as Twenge told me during a discussion about her work, "a celebrity world that showcases narcissism." Indeed, Twenge thinks popular culture has crossed the line and that such narcissistic traits are now viewed and portrayed as a good thing.

To be fair, not everyone agrees about the degree to which narcissism is actually increasing. But, regardless of the magnitude of the phenomenon—and I believe that the data, while still evolving, are pretty darn convincing—the implications could be significant. There is, for example, evidence that the current cohort of youth feels more entitled and is less interested in community and social engagements. (Note: this is not to say *every* youth has this disposition. I know many highly engaged and socially conscience young people!) They crave, more than generations before, extrinsic rewards and aspirations, such as fame, wealth, looks and material possessions, and are less interested in intrinsic rewards. Many studies tell us that a focus on intrinsic goals (such as community, personal growth and relationships) is positively associated with indicators of psychological well-being and that an orientation toward extrinsic life goals is associated with decreased well-being.

All of that being said, we need to take care not to place too much blame on the attractive shoulders of celebrities. There are bigger fish to fry, such as the growing economic disparity found throughout the world. Celebrity culture is a systemic phenomenon. Gwyneth may be a kook, but she didn't create the social and psychological conditions that give celebrity culture its considerable influence. As noted by Sternheimer, celebrity culture is a "collective fantasy." It isn't imposed from above by Gwyneth, Pamela, *People* magazine or the Hollywood elites. It is a force that both mirrors and shapes our hopes and desires, creating the compelling illusion that a transcendent beauty can be acquired and an elevating fame and fortune achieved by all. It seems that we are caught in a big, self-perpetuating celebrity-fueled cycle that goes something like this: declining social mobility and diminishing life options lead to increasing dreams of celebrity fame and fortune. This, in turn, enhances the power and allure of celebrity, which causes a focus (perhaps with an ever-increasing narcissistic resolve) on extrinsic aspirations that leads to less happiness and distracts us (and society more generally) from actions that may enhance social mobility, such as education and advocacy for social change.

It is, I admit, a rather grand claim. But it is not without foundation. As I have tried to show throughout this book, we humans, whether we like it or not, are unusually interested in and influenced by celebrities and celebrity culture. And both the interest and their influence seem to be intensifying. At a minimum, we need to take steps to gain a greater appreciation of the long-term implications of this trend. And, perhaps most importantly, we need to strive, collectively, to put celebrity culture in its proper and entirely worthy place: as a fun and entertaining diversion.

Now someone hand me the latest issue of *People* magazine.

I started this journey through celebrity culture at an *American Idol* audition. I was surrounded by thousands of struggling singers who had the attainment of celebrity status as their primary motive. I had the opportunity to chat with dozens of these individuals. Many of them were making significant sacrifices in order to keep their dream alive. They told me, straight out, that fame was the goal. Did any of them succeed? Did any get even a moment of national TV exposure? Nope. But guess who did?

The week I work on this concluding chapter is the same week, appropriately enough, that the new season of *American Idol* airs. I am excited to see if any of the people I met at the audition made it in front of the judges. I am curious, for example, to see if Shakespeare Sunday will get to perform one of her original songs. Will the woman with pink hair finally get past the first round? Will the hoodie-wearing teenager start her climb out of poverty toward fame and fortune? It is close to midnight when I finally find time to watch the episode I recorded earlier in the evening. It is a two-hour-long show and I am dead tired, so I fast-forward through much of the program, scanning the screen for a familiar face. I see nobody I know. No Shakespeare. No pink hair. No hoodie. But then, near the end of the show, I see a very familiar face sticking out of a crowd. My face! I am on TV for half a second, perhaps less.

I freeze the image. Unlike the jubilant expressions on the young contestants that surround me in the shot, I have an oddly pained look, as if I were drowning and gulping for air. The shock of seeing myself on TV causes me to call out. "I made it on *Idol*! Hey, everyone, I'm on *American Idol*!"

"Shhhhh!" Joanne responds from upstairs. "Don't wake up the house."

"But, but … I'm on *American Idol* …" I say to myself, lamely pointing at the TV screen and my frozen, contorted face.

ACKNOWLEDGMENTS

This book attempts to cover a lot of topics from a wide range of perspectives. I therefore sought input from an eclectic range of academic experts. But I also wanted to move beyond the scientific literature in order to incorporate the views of individuals in the entertainment industry. As such, my first big thank you goes to the many musicians, actors, writers, directors, etc.—some successful, some struggling—who generously gave me their time and insights. Their input was invaluable. Many of these individuals requested anonymity, often because they felt it would allow them to be more frank. The trade-off was worth it, I think. While many did not make it into the pages of this book, their candid stories informed much of my work and analysis.

Special thanks must also go to my good friend Tim Okamura. A renowned painter and a bit of a celebrity in his own right, he connected me to many knowledgeable individuals, acted as an email conduit for some of the interviews (e.g., Munn and Greenberg) and served as a sounding board for my many crazy ideas. Whether my query was about trying out for *Idol* or hanging with porn stars, his advice was always the same: go for it! I would similarly like to thank my brothers, Case and Sean, two of the brightest individuals around. Their constant support, suggestions and encouragement are always hugely appreciated.

I am also deeply indebted to Gwyneth Paltrow. Much of this book was inspired by her musings on health and beauty. Indeed, I thought about structuring the entire book around Gwyneth's antics. But two things changed my mind. First, poor Gwyneth got a lot of flack in 2013 and 2014. She didn't need more hurled in her direction, even if the hurler was an obscure Canadian academic. Second, getting near Gwyneth isn't easy. I tried. Often. I was told by her publicist that Gwyneth "is going to pass" on my interview request (surprise, surprise). I snuck into one of the gyms she owns with Tracy Anderson, but no Gwyneth. I contacted and chatted with several of her friends and acquaintances (all off the record and anonymously … of course). These discussions provided insight but got me no closer. I tried to attend a ceremony in Chicago where Gwyneth was getting an award, but was denied press credentials. Etc. So my plan to have a nice chitchat with Gwyneth on the science of health and fitness never panned out. But please know, Gwyneth, you remain a true inspiration! Perhaps we could have a coffee … er, herbal tea … sometime in the future? Give me a call.

While Gwyneth and I never had the opportunity to hang, I did have the privilege of interviewing and/or interacting with a wonderful assortment of individuals, including a member of the House of Lords (and I interviewed him *in* the House of Lords), world-famous actors, struggling but brilliant musicians, a Hollywood dermatologist, a celebrity physician, *American Idol* contestants, women who work in the adult entertainment business, etc. It has been a unique and enormously entertaining ride. And I am incredibly grateful for these individuals' help.

Without their involvement this book would not have been possible. So, a massive thank you to Annalise Acorn (University of Alberta); Lisa Leuschner Andersen (San Francisco); Pamela Anderson (Vancouver); Alison Arngrim (Hollywood); Moses Avalon (Los Angeles); Katherine Bao (Manhattanville College); Kirk Barber (University of Calgary); Rhonda Bell (University of Alberta); Tanya Berry (University of Alberta); Marie Bertrand (Skin Science); Jessica Biesiekierski (KU Leuven); Arie Benchetrit (plastic surgeon, Montreal); Jennifer Blake (Society of Obstetricians and Gynaecologists of Canada [SOGC]); Susan Blond (New York); Norman Brown (University of Alberta); Joan Chrisler (Connecticut College); LuAnn Claps (New York); Erin Currier (Washington, DC); Chris de Gar (University of Alberta); Bob Demarco (Brooklyn); Stephen Duncombe (NYU); Emme (New York); Nancy Etcoff (Harvard University); The Fabulous Calgary Sisters (producer/writer/lawyer) (Hollywood); Chris Ferguson (Stetson University); Yoni Freedhoff (Bariatric Medical Institute); Howard Steven Friedman (United Nations); Ramesh Ganeshram (New York); Curtis Gillespie (Edmonton); Gary Fisher (University of Michigan); Joshua Gamson (USCA); Peter Gibson (Monash University); Daniel Gilbert (Harvard); Bryan Greenberg (New York); Christopher E.M. Griffiths (University of Manchester); Zach Hambrick (Michigan State University); Daniel S. Hamermesh (University of Texas); Steven Hoffman (McMaster University); Samuel J. Howard-Spink (NYU); A.J. Jacobs (New York); Camilla Knight (Swansea University); Lord Richard Layard (Centre for Economic Performance at the London School of Economics); Lainey Lui (gossip columnist and TV host); Karen Madsen (University of Alberta); Alice E. Marwick (Fordham University); Chris McCabe (University of Alberta); Linda McCarger (University of Alberta); Ben McConnell, former Beach House drummer (album: *Devotion*) (Paris); Mary McDonough; Ashley Mears (Boston University); Tim Monich (everywhere, it seems); Amy Muise (University of Toronto); Olivia Munn (New York); Matthew Nisbet (American University); John O'Callahan (Edmonton); Nan Okun (Maternal Fetal Medicine, Toronto); Dana Olstad (University of Alberta); Chris Peacocke (Edmonton); T.W. Peacocke (Toronto); Tom Peacocke (Edmonton); Ivona Percec (University of Pennsylvania); Paul Petersen (Hollywood); Rebecca Puhl (Yale University); Dhru Purohit (Los Angeles); Kim Raine (University of Alberta); Rhonda Rand (Hollywood); Donna Rockwell (clinical psychologist); Jacques Romney (University of Alberta); David Sarwer (University of Pennsylvania); Jai Shah (McGill University); Tali Sharot (University College London); Emily Shores (McGill); Michael Simkins (London); Jeremy Snyder (SFU); Viren Swami (University of Westminster); James Turnbull (Korea); Leigh Turner (University of Minnesota); Jean Tweng (San Diego State University); Yalda T. Uhls (Children's Digital Media Center LA); Vanessa and Elena ("The Valley"); Walter Willett (Harvard University); and Kyla Wise (Vancouver); all the individuals who requested anonymity (New York and Hollywood); and anyone I forgot!

I also appreciate the continued support and help from my superb colleagues at the University of Alberta and the Health Law Institute, including Melissa Hartley, Ubaka Ogbogu, Maeghan Toews, Kalina Kaminova, Marianne Clarke, Amir Reshef, Erin Nelson, Nicki Baron, Christen Rachul and especially Robyn Hyde-Lay, who delivered a continuous stream of useful research and ideas.

Thanks must also go to my wonderful agents, Chris Bucci and Anne McDermid. They provided much-needed encouragement and advice on scope and tone. I am also deeply indebted to Diane Turbide and the entire team at Penguin Canada for their continued support, and to Jonathan Webb for his outstanding editorial work.

I am thankful to the many funding agencies that have supported my research, including the Canada Research Chairs program, the Trudeau Foundation, the Alberta Heritage Foundation for Medical Research, the Stem Cell Network (National Centres of Excellence), AllerGen (National Centres of Excellence), Genome Alberta, the Canadian Institutes of Health Research, the Social Sciences and Humanities Research Council, the CCSC and the Alberta Policy Coalition for Cancer Prevention.

Finally, my biggest thanks must go to my long-suffering family. One of the themes of this book is that happiness and fulfillment do not come from wealth, material possessions, awards, career success, fame or even recognition from your peers. It comes from simple day-to-day pleasures and, most importantly, from the people with whom you have the closest relationships. In this latter category, I have been truly blessed. So, thank you, Adam, Alison, Jane, Michael and Joanne. You are all superstars.

REFERENCES AND NOTES

The references are organized according to chapter. In the text, I tried to include enough information so that the relevant study could be identified in the alphabetical lists that follow below. For many of the references, I have also added a short description of its relevance. There is a huge amount of literature available, and as such, this is far from comprehensive. Nevertheless, I hope it gives the reader a sense of the work that informed my research. As you will note, material came from a variety of sources, including the popular press and celebrity blogs. The latter gives a sense of how the popular press represents the particular or may have been the source for a quote, etc. It should also be noted that different versions of my experience with the Clean Cleanse and the gluten-free analysis appeared, respectively, in *Eighteen Bridges* and the *Toronto Star*. Finally, I'd like to comment on the challenge of researching celebrity statements, beliefs and actions. Much of this comes from celebrity-focused magazines, blogs and the general pop culture universe. I recognize that these are not necessarily perfect representations of reality. For example, the information may have been altered by a publicist or may be the speculation of a celebrity blogger. But given that the point of the book is to explore the impact of celebrity culture, it is the public face of celebrity that is most relevant.

PREFACE: ARE CELEBRITIES MORE WRONG THAN EVER?

American Society of Clinical Oncology. 2018. *National Cancer Opinion Survey*. October. https://www.asco.org/sites/new-www.asco.org/files/content-files /research-and-progress/documents/2018-NCOS-Results.pdf.

Broniatowski, D.A., et al. 2018. Weaponized health communication: Twitter bots and Russian trolls amplify the vaccine debate. *American Journal of Public Health* 108.

Chotiner, I. 2019. Does democracy need truth?: a conversation with the historian Sophia Rosenfeld. *The New Yorker*, January 31. https:// www.newyorker.com/news/q-and-a/does-democracy-need-truth-a -conversation-with-the-historian-sophia-rosenfeld.

Colagrossi, M. 2019. American kids today dream of being vloggers, not astronauts. Big Think, August 1. https://bigthink.com/culture-religion /vloggers-astronauts.

Dorius, S. et al. 2018. Sowing the seeds of skepticism: Russian state news and anti-GMO sentiment. *GM Crops & Food*, 9:53–58.

Edelman Trust Barameter. 2018. *Global Report*. February. https://www.edelman. com/sites/g/files/aatuss191/files/2018-10/2018_Edelman_Trust_Barometer _Global_Report_FEB.pdf.

Knight Foundation. 2018. *American Views: Trust, Media and Democracy*. January. https://kf-site-production.s3.amazonaws.com/publications/pdfs/000/000 /242/original/KnightFoundation_AmericansViews_Client_Report _010917_Final_Updated.pdf.

Gelles, D. 2019. Gwyneth Paltrow is all business. *New York Times*, March 6. https://www.nytimes.com/2019/03/06/business/gwyneth-paltrow-goop -corner-office.html.

Greenberg, J., et al. 2017. *Vaccine Hesitancy: In Search of the Risk Communication Comfort Zone*. Public Library of Science Current Outbreaks, March. https://www.ncbi.nlm.nih.gov/pubmed/28357154.

Gunter, J. 2018. Don't listen to Gwyneth Paltrow: keep your coffee well away from your rectum. *The Guardian*, January 9. https://www.theguardian.com/commentisfree/2018/jan/09/gwyneth-paltrow-goop-coffee-enema-colonic-irrigation.

Jaschik, S. 2019. Falling confidence in higher ed. Inside Higher Ed, October 9. https://www.insidehighered.com/news/2018/10/09/gallup-survey-finds-falling-confidence-higher-education.

Johnson, S., et al. 2018. Use of alternative medicine for cancer and its impact on survival. 110 *Journal of the National Cancer Institute* 121–124.

Johnson, S., et al. 2018. Complementary medicine, refusal of conventional cancer therapy, and survival among patients with curable cancers. 4 *JAMA Oncology* 1375-1381.

Kirkey, S. A third of Canadians say science on vaccines isn't "quite clear": poll. *National Post*, February 21.

Murphy, G., et al. 2019. False memories for fake news during Ireland's abortion referendum. *Psychological Science* 1–11.

Polage, D. 2012. Making up history: false memories of fake news stories. 8 *Europe's Journal of Psychology* 245–250.

Schomer, A. 2019. Influencer marketing 2019: why brands can't get enough of an $8 billion ecosystem driven by Kardashians, moms, and tweens. *Business Insider*, July 15. https://www.businessinsider.com/the-2019-influencer-marketing-report-2019-7.

Thompson, E. 2019. Poll finds 90% of Canadians have fallen for fake news. CBC News, June 11. https://www.cbc.ca/news/politics/fake-news-facebook-twitter-poll-1.5169916.

Turner, C. 2018. Revealed: top career aspirations for today's primary school children. *The Telegraph*, January 19. https://www.telegraph.co.uk/education/2018/01/19/revealed-top-career-aspirations-todays-primary-school-children/.

van den Brink-Muinen, A., et al. 2006. Does trust in health care influence the use of complementary and alternative medicine by chronically ill people? 6 *BMC Public Health*.

INTRODUCTION: IDOL DREAMS

Ayers, John W. et al. 2014. Do celebrity cancer diagnoses promote primary cancer prevention? *Preventive Medicine* 58:81–4: doi:10.1016/j.yp med.2013.11.007.

BBC News. 2013. "Viewpoint: Did our brains evolve to foolishly follow celebrities?" June 25. www.bbc.co.uk/news/magazine-23046602.

Click, Melissa A. et al. 2013. Making monsters: Lady Gaga, fan identification, and social media. *Popular Music and Society* 36:360–79.

Currid-Halkett, Elizabeth. 1994. *Starstruck: The business of celebrity*. New York: Faber and Faber.

Gamson, Joshua. 1994. *Claims to fame: Celebrity in contemporary America*. Berkeley: University of California Press.

Gross, L.A. 2009. Broken trust: Lessons from the Vaccine–Autism Wars. *PLoSBiol* 7 (7): e1000114: doi:10.1371/journal.pbio.1000114.

Halpern, Jake. 2007. *Fame junkies: The hidden truths behind America's favorite addiction*. Boston: Mariner Books.

Henrich, Joseph, and Francisco J. Gil-White. 2001. The evolution of prestige: Freely conferred deference as a mechanism for enhancing the benefits of cultural transmission. *Evolution and Human Behavior* 22:165–96.

Higgins, Michael. 2013. U.S. infatuation with celebrity lifestyle killing the American dream: Barack Obama. *National Post*, July 31. http://news.nationalpost.com/2013/07/31/u-s-infatuation-with-celebrity-lifestyle-killing-the-american-dream-barack-obama/.

Hoffman, Steven, and C. Tan. 2013. Following celebrities' medical advice: Meta-narrative analysis. *BMJ* 347:f7151. This is a nice review of the evidence surrounding the influence celebrities have of health decisions.

Kamenova, Kalina, Amir Reshef and T. Caulfield. 2013. Angelina Jolie's faulty gene: Newspaper coverage of a celebrity's preventive bilateral mastectomy in Canada, the United States, and the United Kingdom. *Genetics in Medicine* 16 (7):522–8.

Marshal, David, ed. 2006. *The celebrity culture reader*. New York: Routledge.

McCutcheon, Lynn E. et al. 2002. Conceptualization and measurement of celebrity worship. *British Journal of Psychology* 93:67–87.

Niederkrotenthaler, T. et al. 2012. Changes in suicide rates following media reports on celebrity suicide: A meta-analysis. *J Epidemiol Community Health* 66:1037–42.

Payne, Tom. 2009. *Fame: What the classics tell us about our cult of celebrity*. New York: Picador.

Robbins, Alexandra. 2013. Celebrity trend uses nutrients hospitals desperately need. July 29. www.washingtonian.com/articles/people/hot-celebrity-trend-worsens-drug-shortages-that-threaten-babies/#.

Schickel, Richard. 1985. *Intimate strangers: The cult of celebrity in America*. Chicago: Ivan R. Dee.

Smith, Philip J. et al. 2011. Parental delay or refusal of vaccine doses, childhood vaccination coverage at 24 months of age, and the Health Belief Model. *Public Health Rep* 126:135–46.

Sternheimer, Karen. 2011. *Celebrity culture and the American dream*. New York: Routledge.

PART I: THE ILLUSION OF CELEBRITY AUTHORITY

CHAPTER I: DIETING, GWYNETH AND MY CLEANSE

Autier, Philippe et al. 2014. Vitamin D status and ill health: A systematic review. *The Lancet Diabetes & Endocrinology* 2:76–89.

Bahlai C.A. et al. 2010. Choosing organic pesticides over synthetic pesticides may not effectively mitigate environmental risk in soybeans. *PLoS ONE* 5:e11250. This study shows organic pesticides are no better, from an environmental perspective, than synthetic.

Bakalar, Nicholos. 2012. Limits of vitamin D supplements. *New York Times,* December 11. http://well.blogs.nytimes.com/2013/12/11/limits-of-vitamin-d-supplements/. Bakalar writes: "Unfortunately, there is probably no benefit to expect from vitamin D supplementation in normally healthy people."

Basker, Dov. 1992. Comparison of taste quality between organically and conventionally grown fruits and vegetables. *American Journal of Alternative Agriculture* 7:129.

BBC Science & Nature. n.d. The truth about food: The detox diet. www .bbc.co.uk/sn/humanbody/truthaboutfood/young/detox.shtml. This is a summary of the show that debunks detox diets.

Beck, Melinda. 2011. City vs. country: Who is healthier? *The Wall Street Journal*, July 12. http://online.wsj.com/news/articles/SB100014240527 02304793504576434442652581806. This reviews a study showing city dwellers as being healthier than those living in the country.

Biesiekierski, J.R., S.L. Peters and E.D. Newnham. 2013. No effects of gluten in patients with self-reported non-celiac gluten sensitivity after dietary reduction of fermentable, poorly absorbed, short-chain carbohydrates. *Gastroenterology*145:320. This terrific study explores the existence of gluten sensitivity.

Biesiekierski, Jessica R., Jane G. Muir and Peter R. Gibson. 2013. Is gluten a cause of gastrointestinal symptoms in people without celiac disease? *Curr Allergy Asthma Rep* 13:631. In this excellent review of the evidence, the authors write: "Non-celiac gluten sensitivity is an entity awaiting validation, better diagnostic criteria, and, if it does exist, pathogenic mechanisms."

Bosy-Westphal, A. et al. 2013. Effect of weight loss and regain on adipose tissue distribution, composition of lean mass and resting energy expenditure in young overweight and obese adults. *Int J Obes* 37:1371. The study did *not* find that yo-yo dieting had an impact on fat distribution, but it did find that it slowed the metabolism that may contribute to weight regain.

Bourn, Diane, and John Prescott. 2002. A comparison of the nutritional value, sensory qualities, and food safety of organically and conventionally produced foods. *Crit Rev Food Sci Nutr* 42:1. This review found no health benefits to organic food.

Callahan, Erica. 2013. Changes in weight loss and lipid profiles after a dietary purification program: A prospective case series. *J Chiropr Med* 12:30. One of the few studies on detox diets, it includes seven subjects and no comparator group.

Casazza, Krista et al. 2013. Myths, presumptions, and facts about obesity. *N Engl J Med* 368:2236.

CBC News. 2014. "Pesticide residue found on nearly half of organic produce" January 8. www.cbc.ca/news/canada/manitoba/pesticide-residue-found -on-nearly-half-of-organic-produce-1.2487712. This is a news report on government data.

Cereda, Emanuele et al. 2011. Weight cycling is associated with body weight excess and abdominal fat accumulation: A cross-sectional study. *Clin Nutr* 30:718. This studies the impact of dieting on fat accumulation.

Champeau, Rachel. 2013. Changing gut bacteria through diet affects brain function, UCLA study shows. *UCLA Newsroom,* May 28. http:// newsroom.ucla.edu/portal/ucla/changing-gut-bacteria-through-245617 .aspx. This proof of concept study explores the link between gut bacteria and brain function.

Clemens, Roger, and Peter Pressman. 2005. Detox diets provide empty promises. *Food Technology* 59:18. It includes a quote on the absurdity of detox diets.

Cohen, Marc. 2007. "Detox": Science or sales pitch? *Aust Fam Physician* 36:1009.

Danhof-Pont, Marie Bernardine et al. 2010. Biomarkers in burnout: A systematic review. *J Psychosom Res* 70:505. The authors write: "No potential biomarkers for burnout were found, largely due to the incom-parability of studies."

DeBenedette, Valerie. 2013. Eating fruits and vegetables tied to longer life. Reuters, July 11. www.reuters.com/article/2013/07/11/us-health-fruits -longer-life-idUSBRE96A0HL20130711. This story is on the study that explored the health value of fruits and veggies.

DiMeglio, D.P., and R.D. Mattes. 2000. Liquid versus solid carbohydrate: Effects on food intake and body weight. *Int J Obes* 24:794. The study showed that increased BMI and calorie intake was associated with the consumption of liquids.

Dye, Christopher. 2008. Health and urban living. *Science* 319:766.

Eberhardt, Mark S., and Elsie R. Pamuk. 2004. The importance of place of residence: Examining health in rural and nonrural areas. *Am J Public Health* 94:1682.

Elli, L. 2012. Where's the evidence for gluten sensitivity? *BMJ* 345:e7360.

Eskine, Kendall J. 2012. Wholesome foods and wholesome morals? Organic foods reduce prosocial behavior and harshen moral judgments. *Soc Psychol Personal Sci* 4:251. This study suggests that buying organic actually makes people less "moral" and altruistic.

FDA. 2011. *Consumer health information: A glimpse at "gluten-free" food labeling*. August. www.fda.gov/downloads/ForConsumers/ConsumerUpdates/UCM266206.pdf.

Fillion, Laurence, and Stacey Arazi. 2002. Does organic food taste better? A claim substantiation approach. *Nutrition & Food Science* 32:153. This study concluded that the "global claim that 'organic food tastes better' is not valid, and each product type should be treated separately before a claim can be made."

Fond, Guillaume et al. 2013. Fasting in mood disorders: Neurobiology and effectiveness. A review of the literature. *Psychiatry Research* 209:253–58. This outlines the psychological effects of fasting/starvation.

Food Standard Agency. 2009. *Comparison of putative health effects of organically and conventionally produced foodstuffs: A systematic review*. Food Standards Agency. http://multimedia.food.gov.uk/multimedia/pdfs/organicreviewreport.pdf. This UK study concluded that there was no health benefit to organic food.

Forman, Joel, and Janet Silverstein. 2012. Organic foods: Health and environmental advantages and disadvantages. *Pediatrics* 130:e1406.

Furlan, A.D. et al. 2005. Acupuncture and dry-needling for low back pain. Cochrane Database Syst Rev CD001351. See more at: http://summaries.cochrane.org/CD001351/acupuncture-and-dry-needling-for-low-back-pain#sthash.lKyvvIWF.dpuf.

Gaesser, Glenn A., and Siddhartha S. Angadi. 2012. Gluten-free diet: Imprudent dietary advice for the general population? *J Acad Nutr Diet* 112:1330. This is a nice summary of the evidence associated with gluten-free diets.

Garth, Ina et al. 2011. Effect of two different weight loss rates on body composition and strength and power related performance in elite athletes. *Int J Sport Nutr Exerc Metab* 21:97. This is a Norwegian study on muscle mass post-fast and with slow weight loss.

Gilsenan, C. et al. 2012. Do organic cherry vine tomatoes taste better than conventional cherry vine tomatoes? A sensory and instrumental comparative study from Ireland. *Journal of Culinary Science & Technology* 10:154.

Hamzaoui-Essoussi, Leila, and Mehdi Zahaf. 2012. Canadian organic food consumers' profile and their willingness to pay premium prices. *Journal of International Food & Agribusiness Marketing* 24:1. The article outlines why people purchase organic food, including the fact that it is part of an alternative lifestyle.

Holmes, Geoffrey. 2013. Non coeliac gluten sensitivity. *Gastroenterol Hepatol Bed Bench* 6:115. This is a review of the issue, including estimates of size of market, etc.

Hormone Health Network. 2010. Adrenal fatigue. www.hormone.org/hormones-and-health/myth-vs-fact. This is a statement from the Network about the evidence surrounding adrenal fatigue.

Houchins, J.A. et al. 2013. Effects of fruit and vegetable, consumed in solid vs beverage forms. *Int J Obes* 37:1109.

Institute of Medicine. 2010. *Dietary reference intakes for calcium and vitamin D.* Institute of Medicine, November 30. http://www.iom.edu/Reports/2010/Dietary-Reference-Intakes-for-Calcium-and-Vitamin-D.aspx.

Jebb, S.A. et al. 1991. Effects of weight cycling caused by intermittent dieting on metabolic rate and body composition in obese women. *Int J Obes* 15:367. This study found no evidence that yo-yo dieting impacted metabolism.

Johnson, Timothy V., Ammara Abbasi and Viraj A. Master. 2013. Systematic review of the evidence of a relationship between chronic psychosocial stress and C-reactive protein. *Mol Diagn Ther* 17:147.

Jones, L.V. et al. 2013. Solid versus liquid: Satiety study in well-adjusted lap-band patients. *Obes Surg* 23:1266.

Junger, Alejandro. 2011. Dr. Junger's recommended blood tests. Clean Program. http://cleanprogram.com/media/files/blood-tests.pdf.

Lee, Jung Sun et al. 2010. Weight loss and regain and effects on body composition: The health, aging, and body composition study. *J Gerontol A Biol*

Sci Med Sci 65:78. This study found that yo-yo dieting "may contribute to a net loss of lean mass in older men but warrants further studies."

Magkos, Faidon et al. 2003. Organic food: Nutritious food or food for thought? A review of the evidence. *Int J Food Sci Nutr* 54:357. The authors write: "Although there is little evidence that organic and conventional foods differ in respect to the concentrations of the various micronutrients (vitamins, minerals and trace elements), there seems to be a slight trend towards higher ascorbic acid content in organically grown leafy vegetables and potatoes."

Mann, Traci et al. 2007. Medicare's search for effective obesity treatments: Diets are not the answer. *Am Psychol* 62:220. This study highlights the ineffectiveness of virtually all diets.

Mason, Caitlin et al. 2013. History of weight cycling does not impede future weight loss or metabolic improvements in postmenopausal women. *Metabolism* 62:127. The history of yo-yo dieting did not impair metabolism of future weight loss.

Mattei, J., S. Bhupathiraju and K.L. Tucker. 2013. Higher adherence to a diet score based on American Heart Association recommendations is associated with lower odds of allostatic load and metabolic syndrome in Puerto Rican adults. *J Nutr* 143:1753.

Maugh II, Thomas H. 2010. Endocrinologists speak out about two "Internet diseases": Adrenal fatigue and Wilson's temperature fatigue. *Los Angeles Times*, September 15. http://articles.latimes.com/2010/sep/15/news/la-heb-internet-diseases-20100915.

Michels, Nathalie et al. 2013. Relation between salivary cortisol as stress biomarker and dietary pattern in children. *Psychoneuroendocrinology* 38:1512.

Mishori, Ranit et al. 2011. The dangers of colon cleansing. *J Fam Practice* 60:454. This paper outlines the lack of evidence to support the use of colon cleanses, etc.

Nackers, Lisa M. et al. 2010. The association between rate of initial weight loss and long-term success in obesity treatment: Does slow and steady win the race? *Int J Behav Med* 17:161.

————. 2013. Effects of prescribing 1,000 versus 1,500 kilocalories per day in the behavioral treatment of obesity: A randomized trial. *Obesity* 21:248.

Nestle, Marion, and Malden C. Nesheim. 2013. To supplement or not to supplement: The U.S. Preventive Services Task Force recommendations on calcium and vitamin D. *Ann Intern Med* 158:701. This is a useful commentary on the recommendations.

Newmaster, S.G. et al. 2013. DNA barcoding detects contamination and substitution in North American herbal products. *BMC Med* 11:222. This study highlights the poor quality of most supplements.

Ng, Serena, and Jonathan Rockoff. 2013. With top lines drooping, firms reach for vitamins. *The Wall Street Journal*, March 31. http://online .wsj.com/news/articles/SB100014241278873243928045783620736 24344816. The authors note that big pharmaceutical companies have purchased supplement companies and that the industry is worth approximately $23 million in the US alone.

Novella, Steven. 2014. Non-celiac gluten sensitivity. *Neurologica* (May 15). In this example of a skeptical look at NCGS, the author concludes: "NCGS is probably not a real entity."

Offit, Paul. 2013. The vitamin myth: Why we think we need supplements. *The Atlantic* (July 19). www.theatlantic.com/health/archive/2013/07/ the-vitamin-myth-why-we-think-we-need-supplements/277947/. This is a terrific piece on the lack of evidence to support the use of vitamins.

Osborn, Robyn L. et al. 2011. Yo-yo dieting in African American women: Weight cycling and health. *Ethnicity & Disease* 21:274. The authors write: "African American women are at risk for weight cycling and it may be associated with greater weight and poorer measures of psychological health."

Preidt, Robert. 2013. No sign that vitamin D supplements help aging bones: Study. *Healthday*, October 10. http://consumer.healthday.com/ bone-and-joint-information-4/osteo-arthritis-news-42/no-sign-that -vitamin-d-supplements-help-aging-bones-study-681008.html. This is a news report on a study in *The Lancet*.

Reid, Ian R., Mark J. Bolland and Andrew Grey. 2013. Effects of vitamin D supplements on bone mineral density: A systematic review and meta-analysis. *The Lancet* 383:136–55. This study shows limited or no benefit to vitamin D in the context of bone health.

Reyes, Naomi R. et al. 2012. Similarities and differences between weight loss maintainers and regainers: A qualitative analysis. *J Acad Nutr Diet* 112:499. This emphasizes the need for continued motivation and lifestyle change.

Rodin, J. et al. 1990. Weight cycling and fat distribution. *Int J Obes* 14:303. This study found that yo-yo dieting did have an impact on fat distribution.

Roeder, Amy. 2013. Skip the juice, go for whole fruit: Eating whole fruits, particularly blueberries, grapes, apples, linked to lower risk of type 2 diabetes. *Harvard Gazette*, August 29. http://news.harvard.edu/gazette/story/2013/08/reduce-type-2-diabetes-risk/.

Romans, S., M. Cohen and T. Forte. 2011. Rates of depression and anxiety in urban and rural Canada. *Soc Psychiatry and Psychiatr Epidemiol* 46:567. This study found lower risk of depression in rural settings.

Rundle, Andrew et al. 2012. Association of childhood obesity with maternal exposure to ambient air polycyclic aromatic hydrocarbons during pregnancy. *Am J Epidemiol* 175:1163. This study linked pollution with obesity.

Sánchez-Villegas, Almudena et al. 2012. Fast-food and commercial baked goods consumption and the risk of depression. *Public Health Nutr* 15:424.

Sarlio-LaÈhteenkorva, S. et al. 2000. A descriptive study of weight loss maintenance: 6 and 15 year follow-up of initially overweight adults. *Int J Obes* 24:116.

Simon, Stacy. 2013. Omega-3 fatty acids linked to increase in prostate cancer risk. *Cancer* (July 17). www.cancer.org/cancer/news/omega-3-fatty-acids-linked-to-increase-in-prostate-cancer-risk.

Singh, G.K. et al. 2013. All-cause and cause-specific mortality among U.S. youth: Socioeconomic and rural–urban disparities and international patterns. *J Urban Health* 90:388. This study showed rural youth were at greater risk.

Singh, Gopal K., and Mohammad Siahpush. 2014. Widening rural–urban disparities in life expectancy, U.S., 1969–2009. *Am J Prev Med* 46:e19–e29. The authors write: "Life expectancy was inversely related to levels of rurality."

Smith-Spangler, Crystal et al. 2012. Are organic foods safer or healthier than conventional alternatives?: A systematic review. *Ann Intern Med* 157:348. This Stanford study found no nutritional difference between organic and conventional foods.

Spence, Des. 2013. Bad medicine: Food intolerance. *BMJ* 346:f529. This editorial notes the role of the profit motive in the gluten-free fad.

Stevens, Victoria L. et al. 2012. Weight cycling and mortality in a large prospective U.S. study. A*m J Epidemiol* 175:785. The authors write: "These results do not support an increased risk of mortality associated with weight cycling [yo-yo dieting]."

Strom, Stephanie. 2012. Has "organic" been oversized? *New York Times*, July 7. www.nytimes.com/2012/07/08/business/organic-food-purists -worry-about-big-companies-influence.html. This story outlines the degree to which the organic food industry has been taken over by "Big Food" companies.

Stubbs, Amy. 2013. Diet heavy in fruits, vegetables protects mental health, while fast food may invite depression: Finland study. *National Post*, September 19. http://life.nationalpost.com/2013/09/19/diet -heavy-in-fruits-vegetables-protects-mental-health-while-fast-food-may -invite-depression-finland-study/. This story is about the study.

Talavera Bianchi, Jose Martin. 2009. Sensory analysis of pacchoi and tomato grown under organic and conventional systems. PhD diss., Kansas State University. The authors write: "There do not appear to be major sensory differences between organic and conventional products specific to the crops and seasons studied."

Theodoratou, Evropi et al. 2014. Vitamin D and multiple health outcomes: Umbrella review of systematic reviews and meta-analyses of observational studies and randomised trials. *BMJ* 348:g2035. This is another study highlighting the equivocal nature of vitamin D evidence. The authors write: "highly convincing evidence of a clear role of vitamin D does not exist for any outcome."

Tomiyama, A. Janet et al. 2010. Low calorie dieting increases cortisol. *Psychosom Med* 72:357.

Tryon, M.S., R. DeCant and K.D. Laugero. 2013. Having your cake and eating it too: A habit of comfort food may link chronic social stress exposure and acute stress-induced cortisol hyporesponsiveness. *Physiol Behav* 32:114–15.

Tsivgoulis, Georgios et al. 2013. Adherence to a Mediterranean diet and risk of incident cognitive impairment. *Neurology* 80:1684.

Tuff, Alice, and Harriet Bell. 2009. The Voice of Young Science network brings you … The detox dossier. *Voice of Young Science.* www.senseaboutscience .org/data/files/resources/48/Detox-Dossier-Embargoed-until-0001 -5th-jan-2009.pdf.

UEF. 2009. Diet is associated with the risk of depression. www.uef.fi/fi/-/ diet-is-associated-with-the-risk-of-depression.

Ulbricht, Catherine et al. 2012. Caffeine clinical bottom line: An evidence-based systematic review by the Natural Standard Research Collaboration. *Alternative and Complementary Therapies* 18:324. This paper provides a nice review of research on the benefits of coffee, including noting the lack of evidence for the use of caffeine to treat wrinkles and cellulite.

Vanga, Rohini, and Daniel A. Leffler. 2013. Gluten sensitivity: Not celiac and not certain. *Gastroenterology* 145:276. This editorial questions the existence of non-celiac gluten sensitivity.

Vlahov, D., S. Galea and N. Freudenberg. 2005. The urban health "Advantage. *J Urban Health* 82:1.

Wallner, S.J. et al. 2004. Body fat distribution of overweight females with a history of weight cycling. *Int J Obes* 28:1143–8. This study finds different fat distribution in women with a history of weight cycling.

Watson, Elaine. 2012. Gluten free "most popular approach to weight loss" for 2013 (but it doesn't work, say dietitians). *Food Navigator*, December 20. www.foodnavigator-usa.com/Markets/Gluten-free-most-popular

-approach-to-weight-loss-for-2013-but-it-doesn-t-work-say-dietitians. This reports on the popularity of gluten free.

White, Bonnie A. et al. 2013. Many apples a day keep the blues away: Daily experiences of negative and positive affect and food consumption in young adults. *Br J Health Psychol* 18:782. This is about the impact of fruits and vegetables on mental health.

Wing, Rena R. et al. 1995. A prospective study of effects of weight cycling on cardiovascular risk factors. *Arch Intern Med* 155:1416.

CHAPTER 2: BEAUTY TIPS FROM BEAUTIFUL PEOPLE

Armstrong, B. et al. 2009. A review of human carcinogens—Part D: Radiation. *The Lancet Oncol* 10:751. This notes the WHO classification of tanning beds as a carcinogen.

Aubin, Henri-Jean. 2012. Weight gain in smokers after quitting cigarettes: Meta-analysis. *BMJ* 345:e4439.

Axelsson, John et al. 2010. Beauty sleep: Experimental study on the perceived health and attractiveness of sleep-deprived people. *BMJ* 341:c6614.

Barsh, Gregory, and Laura D. Attardi. 2007. A healthy tan? *N Engl J Med* 356:2208.

Basch, Corey Hannah et al. 2012. Improving understanding about tanning behaviors in college students. *J Am Coll Health* 60:250. This is a referenced study about college students' practices and attitudes.

BBC. 2013. "Sleep 'boosts brain cell numbers.'" *BBC News Health*, September 3. www.bbc.co.uk/news/health-23932577.

Bergamin, Elaina et al. 2013. Trends in tobacco and alcohol brand placements in popular U.S. movies, 1996 through 2009. *JAMA Pediatr* 167:634.

Bures, Frank. 2012. Be skeptical of skin product claims. *Winona Daily News*, February 5. www.winonadailynews.com/news/connections/article_1a7b4884-4eb7-11e1-b37c-001871e3ce6c.html. The author quotes Dr. Gold on the questionable value of expensive moisturizers, specifically a $700 moisturizer.

Cappuccio, F.P. et al. 2010. Sleep duration and all-cause mortality: A systematic review and meta-analysis of prospective studies. *SLEEP* 33:585.

CBC Community Team. 2011. Do health spas need more strict regulations? *Your Community Blog*, July 30. www.cbc.ca/newsblogs/your community/2011/07/do-health-spas-need-more-strict-regulations.html.

CBC News. 2012. "5 facts on tanning and skin cancer." *CBC News*, April 25. www.cbc.ca/news/health/story/2012/04/25/melanoma-skin-cancer -tanning.html.

CDC. 2011. *Insufficient sleep is a public health epidemic*. Centers for Disease Control and Prevention. www.cdc.gov/features/dssleep/. This is a review of research on sleep behavior in the US.

Charlesworth, A. 2005. Smoking in the movies increases adolescent smoking: A review. *Pediatrics* 116:1516.

Chen, N. et al. 2010. Acupuncture for Bell's palsy. Cochrane Database Syst Rev CD002914. This is an example of a review that outlines the poor evidence-base surrounding acupuncture.

Chiolero, Arnaud et al. 2008. Consequences of smoking for body weight, body fat distribution, and insulin resistance. *Am J Clin Nutr* 87:801. This is a good review of the impact of smoking on body weight. It refers to a paper showing that, over time, smokers and nonsmokers gain about the same amount of weight.

Clarke, Laura Hurd, and Alexandra Korotchenko. 2009. Older women and suntanning: The negotiation of health and appearance risks. *Sociology Health Illn* 31:748.

Colquhoun, David, and Steven P. Novella. 2013. Acupuncture is theatrical placebo. *Anesthesia and Analgesia* 116:1360–63. This is a skeptical analysis of acupuncture.

Craymer, Lucy. 2012. Latest skin-care buzz: Bee venom. *The Wall Street Journal*, June 27. http://online.wsj.com/article/SB10001424052702303 649504577492801088949864.html. This is one of the few media articles that questions the efficacy of bee venom as an anti-aging treatment.

Cunningham, Kate. 2011. What credit crunch? Women splash £133k on chasing perfection. *Express*, February 21. www.express.co.uk/news/ uk/230289/What-credit-crunch-Women-splash-133k-on-chasing -perfection. The amount is over US $200,000.

Daily News 2013. Placenta face mask tops list of anti-aging treatments for women. *Daily News*, July 5. www.nydailynews.com/life-style/placenta -face-mask-anti-aging-article-1.1390885. This reports on a survey about what kind of anti-aging products U.K. women use.

Dixon, Helen et al. 2008. Portrayal of tanning, clothing fashion and shade use in Australian women's magazines, 1987–2005. *Health Educ Res* 23:791.

Donoyama, N. et al. 2012. Cosmetic acupuncture to enhance facial skin appearance: A preliminary study. *Acupuncture in Medicine* 30:152.

Doyle, Kathryn. 2014. Tobacco on TV tied to adult smoking rates. Reuters News, April 15. www.reuters.com/article/2014/04/15/us-tv-tobacco -rates-idUSBREA3E1IA20140415. This is a news report of a study exploring the impact of TV on smoking behavior.

Dumas, Daisy. 2011. So that's her secret! Gwyneth Paltrow reveals her favourite anti-ageing beauty trick—and at $185, it doesn't come cheap. *Mail Online*, July 29. www.dailymail.co.uk/femail/article-2020014/ Gwyneth-Paltrow-reveals-beauty-anti-ageing-secrets-185-theyre-cheap .html. This is an example of a Gwyneth Paltrow media quote on sonic sea serum treatment.

Edmonton Journal. 2013. Snails—all in the line of beauty. *Edmonton Journal*, July 19. www2.canada.com/edmontonjournal/news/story .html?id=345b0b5a-22fc-4195-af5a-bf302c1512c7.

Elliott, Anthony. 2011. "I want to look like that!": Cosmetic surgery and celebrity culture. *Cultural Sociology* 5:463. This article is on the role of celebrity culture in shaping attitudes toward beauty and, in particular, cosmetic surgery.

Ericson, John. 2013. Time for beauty rest: Skin aging linked to lack of sleep. *Medical Daily*, July 23. www.medicaldaily.com/articles/17705/20130723/sleep -aging-skin-beauty-rest-estee-lauder.htm. This article summarizes studies on the benefits of sleep, including recent data on its impact on aging.

Fisher, Gary J. et al. 2008. Looking older: Fibroblast collapse and therapeutic implications. *Arch Dermatol* 144:666. This is a terrific review of the evidence around anti-aging therapies.

Fogel, Joshua, and Faye Krausz. 2013. Watching reality television beauty shows is associated with tanning lamp use and outdoor tanning among college students. *J Am Acad Dermatol* 68:785.

Goldstein, Jacob. 2008. Slim evidence for effectiveness of cellulite treatments. *The Wall Street Journal Health Blog*, August 19. http://blogs.wsj.com/health/2008/08/19/slim-evidence-for-effectiveness-of-cellulite-treatments/. Robert A. Weiss, the former president of the American Society for Dermatologic Surgery, is quoted as saying: "There's nothing that has been shown in any objective way to create improvement for cellulite."

Grether-Beck, S. et al. 2008. Bioactive molecules from the Blue Lagoon: In vitro and in vivo assessment of silica mud and microalgae extracts for their effects on skin barrier function and prevention of skin ageing, *Exp Dermatol* 17:771.

Helfrich, Yolanda R. et al. 2007. Effect of smoking on aging of photoprotected skin. *Arch Dermatol* 143:397. Among other things, this study demonstrates that "the degree of photoprotected skin aging correlates well with age and packs of cigarettes smoked per day."

Holman, Dawn M., and Meg Watson. 2013. Correlates of intentional tanning among adolescents in the United States: A systematic review of the literature. *J Adolesc Health* 52:s52. This study finds that wanting to look like a celebrity is associated with tanning behavior.

Howard, H. et al. 2010. Incidence estimate of nonmelanoma skin cancer in the United States, 2006. *Arch Dermatol* 146:283.

Hruza, G. et al. 2009. Skin rejuvenation and wrinkle reduction using a fractional radiofrequency system. *J Drugs Dermatol* 8:259.

Hughes, Maria Celia B. et al. 2013. Sunscreen and prevention of skin aging: A randomized trial. *Ann Intern Med* 158:781. This is a study on the anti-aging benefits of sunscreen.

Humbert, Philippe et al. 2011. Beauty from inside: Nutrition-based strategies in cosmetic dermatology. In *Nutrition for healthy skin: Strategies for clinical and cosmetic practice*, ed. Jean Krutmann and Philippe Humbert, 189–96. Berlin: Springer. This offers a perspective on the benefits of good nutrition for healthy skin.

REFERENCES AND NOTES

Imaging Excellence from Canfield. n.d. VISIA Complexion Analysis Machine. Imaging Excellence from Canfield. www.canfieldsci.com/ Imaging_Systems/Products/VISIA/VISIA_FAQ.html. This website states that the facial assessment machine is used as a "sales tool to promote their Olay and SKII brands of cosmetic products." See also: Imaging Excellence from Canfield. VISIA Complexion Analysis. Imaging Excellence from Canfield. www.canfieldsci.com/imaging_systems/facial_ systems/VISIA_Complexion_Analysis.html.

Institute of Medicine. 2004. Report sets dietary intake levels for water, salt, and potassium to maintain health and reduce chronic disease risk. The National Academies, February 11. www8.nationalacademies.org/ onpinews/newsitem.aspx?RecordID=10925.

Institute of Medicine. 2005. *Dietary reference intakes for water, potassium, sodium, chloride, and sulfate.* Washington, DC: The National Academies Press. http://books.nap.edu/openbook.php?record_id=10925. This is a report on the amount of water required. See also the press release with a relevant quote: www8.nationalacademies.org/onpinews/newsitem .aspx?RecordID=10925.

International SPA Association. 2011. International SPA Association releases 2011 U.S. spa industry study. *International Spa Association*, October 4. www.experienceispa.com/articles/index.cfm?action=view&articleID=507. This is an example of industry stats on the size of the spa industry and the number of spa visits.

Jablonski, Nina G. 2010. From Bardot to Beckham: The decline of celebrity. *Skin Cancer Foundation* 28:42–4. www.skincancer.org/prevention/ tanning/from-bardot-to-beckham-the-decline-of-celebrity-tanning. This article reviews the nature and impact of the celebrity-inspired rise of suntanning behaviors. It also notes that some celebs, like Victoria Beckham, are becoming more responsible.

Khan, Misbah H. et al. 2010. Treatment of cellulite. *Am Acad Dermatol* 62:373. This is a great review of the relevant science.

Koh, Suna, Joanne Jung-EunYoo and Carl A. Boger Jr. 2010. Importance-performance analysis with benefit segmentation of spa goers. *International Journal of Contemporary Hospitality Management* 22:718. This reports on the size and nature of the spa market (e.g., annual revenue of approximately $10 billion).

Latreille, Julie et al. 2012. Dietary monounsaturated fatty acids intake and risk of skin photoaging. *PLoS ONE* 7:e44490.

London, Bianca. 2013. Could a cream made of COFFEE BEANS banish cellulite? *Mail Online*, April 26. www.dailymail.co.uk/femail/article-2315203/Coffee-bean-cellulite-cream-Slimming-Coffee-Cream -Brazil-claims-banish-cellulite-orange-peel-free-skin.html. This is an example of a media article talking about the new (and bogus) coffee bean cure.

————. 2013. The leather effect: One in five Brits regret sunbathing in their youth ... and nearly 40% blame their PARENTS. *The Daily Mail*, June 18. www.dailymail.co.uk/femail/article-2350900/The-leather-effect-One -Brits-regret-sunbathing-youth--nearly-40-blame-PARENTS.html. This is not the best source and the study was supported by industry. The survey was tied to a campaign to support use of sunscreen co-sponsored by the British Skin Foundation. (See also http://your.asda.com/press-centre/ don-t-get-burnt.)

————. 2013. Gwyneth Paltrow, 40, reveals the secret to her lean body (and how naughty weekend treats of cigarettes and red wine keep her "vibrant"). *Mail Online*, July 29. www.dailymail.co.uk/femail/ article-2380776/Gwyneth-Paltrow-How-stay-slim-like-Star-40-shares -secrets-maintaining-lean-body.html.

Maier-Schwartz, Sagit. 2013. Bringing Beverly Hills cosmetic surgery to the Middle East. *The Atlantic*, May 29. www.theatlantic.com/health/ archive/2013/05/bringing-beverly-hills-cosmetic-surgery-to-the-middle -east/276302/.

Makrantonaki, Evgenia. 2012. Genetics and skin aging. *Dermatoendocrinol* 4:280. This is a nice review on the role of genes and ethnicity in the context of skin.

Makrantonaki, Evegenia et al. 2012. Identification of biomarkers of human skin ageing in both genders. Wnt signalling: A label of skin ageing? *PLoS ONE* 7:e50393. This paper looks at the existence of biomarkers to predict aging.

REFERENCES AND NOTES

Marrett, Loraine D. et al. 2010. Work-time sun behaviors among Canadian outdoor workers: Results from the 2006 National Sun Survey. *Can J Public Health* 101:I19. This study shows that less than 30% of outdoor workers wear sunscreen.

Marszal, Andrew. 2013. Mad Men boost for Lucky Strike cigarettes angers campaigners. *The Telegraph*, September 22. www.telegraph.co.uk/health/healthnews/10326252/Mad-Men-boost-for-Lucky-Strike-cigarettes-angers-campaigners.html.

Mayes, Andrew E. et al. 2010. Environmental and lifestyle factors associated with perceived facial age in Chinese women. *PLoS ONE* 5:e15270. This study shows the impact of environmental factors on aging.

Mayo Clinic. 2014. Cellulite. www.mayoclinic.com/health/cellulite/DS00891.

Meng, Juan, and Po-Lin Pan. 2012. Investigating the effects of cosmeceutical product advertising in beauty-care decision making. *International Journal of Pharmaceutical and Healthcare Marketing* 6:250. This is a study on how women make decisions about anti-aging products. It also notes the size of the global market as over $27 billion in 2010.

Metro. 2013. Japanese beauty clinic offering "snail facial." *Metro*, July 14. http://metro.co.uk/2013/07/14/japanese-beauty-clinic-offering-snail-facial-3881939/. This article includes a quote on snail facial.

Mitteness, Phillip. 2013. Anti-aging: The trends and challenges in new product development. *GCI*, August 6. www.gcimagazine.com/marketstrends/segments/skincare/Anti-Aging-The-Trends-and-Challenges-in-New-Product-Development-218560461.html. The article estimates that the global anti-aging market will be $291 billion by 2015.

Moses, S.W. et al. 2006. The Dead Sea: A unique natural health resort. *IMAJ* 8:483–8. This paper reviews data on benefits of natural climatotherapy at the Dead Sea.

Muckelbauer, Rebecca et al. 2013. Association between water consumption and body weight outcomes: A systematic review. *Am J Clin Nutr* 98:282. This is a study on the impact of water on weight loss.

Muise, Amy, and Serge Desmarais. 2010. Women's perceptions and use of "anti-aging" products. *Sex Roles* 63:126.

Nagata, Chisato et al. 2010. Association of dietary fat, vegetables and antioxidant micronutrients with skin ageing in Japanese women. *Br J Nutr* 103:1493.

Neill, Ushma S. 2012. Skin care in the aging female: Myths and truths. *J Clin Invest* 122:473. This is a terrific review of evidence associated with anti-aging treatments. The article notes, for example, several experts who feel spa facials do more harm than good.

Nolan, Katherine, and Ellen Marmur. 2012. Over-the-counter topical skincare products: A review of the literature. *J Drugs Dermatol* 11:220.

Osterhout, Jacob E. 2013. Seeking a royal sniffer: New York women rushing to get the Kate Middleton nose. *Daily News*, March 13. www.nydailynews.com/life-style/ny-women-rushing-kate-middleton-nose-article-1.1287848#ixzz2cLexhR6L.

Patel, S.R. 2009. Reduced sleep as an obesity risk factor. *Obes Rev* 10:61. This study shows that "reduced sleep appears to represent a novel, independent risk factor for increased weight gain."

Pitak-Arnnop, Poramate et al. 2011. Gold for facial skin care: Fact or fiction? *Aesth Plast Surg* 35:1184. This is a nice review of much of the literature on common cosmeceutical ingredients, including gold.

Poensin, Dominique et al. 2003. Effects of mud pack treatment on skin microcirculation. *Joint Bone Spine* 70:367. This small study suggests that mudpacks might help with joint pain.

Potter, Beth et al. 2004. Does a relationship exist between body weight, concerns about weight, and smoking among adolescents? *Nicotine Tob Res* 6:397.

Quan, Taihao et al. 2011. Retinoids suppress cysteine-rich protein 61 (CCN1), a negative regulator of collagen homeostasis, in skin equivalent cultures and aged human skin in vivo. *Exp Dermatol* 20:572. The authors write: "Vitamin A and its metabolites have been shown to improve chronologically aged and photoaged skin by promoting deposition of new collagen and preventing its degradation."

Reynolds, Gretchen. 2014. Younger skin through exercise. *The New York Times*, April 16. http://well.blogs.nytimes.com/2014/04/16/younger-skin-through-exercise/?_php=true&_type=blogs&_r=0. This article reports on McMaster University research on the impact of exercise on skin health.

Rose, Les. 2013. Do further studies on acupuncture for pain make sense? An informal review. *Focus Altern Complement Ther* 18:85. This study shows that the effect size for acupuncture studies is small.

Sabanayagam, C., and A. Shankar. 2010. Sleep duration and cardiovascular disease: Results from the National Health Interview Survey. *SLEEP* 33:1037. This is an example of a study on the importance of sleep in the context of cardiovascular disease.

Sachs, D.L., and J.J. Voorhees. 2011. Age-reversing drugs and devices in dermatology. *Clin Pharmacol Ther* 89:34. This is a great review of what works, which is not much. For example, the authors note: "In general, oral supplementation with antioxidants has not been shown to be effective in improving photoaged skin."

Saskatchewan Cancer Agency. 2011. Skin cancer prevention. www. saskcancer.ca/Background%20Document. This offers statistics on sunscreen use, etc.

Shadel, William G. et al. 2013. Exposure to pro-smoking media in college students: Does type of media channel differentially contribute to smoking risk? *Ann Behav Med* 45:387.

Sidorsky, Tivon, and Lionel Bercovitch. 2012. Spa, MD: When dermatology meets aromatherapy. In *Dermatoethics: Contemporary Ethics and Professionalism in Dermatology*, ed. Lionel Bercovitch and Clifford Perlis, 157. London: Springer. This article notes that there is little regulation of spas in the US.

Sies, H., and W. Stahl. 2004. Nutritional protection against skin damage from sunlight. *Annu Rev Nutr* 24:173.

Simon, Harvey. 2012. Skin wrinkles and blemishes. University of Maryland Medical Center. http://umm.edu/health/medical/reports/articles/skin-wrinkles-and-blemishes. Excellent summary of the cause, prevention and treatment of wrinkles.

Stamford, Nicholas P. 2012. Stability, transdermal penetration, and cutaneous effects of ascorbic acid and its derivatives. *J Cosmet Dermatol* 11:310.

The Telegraph. 2013. Unhealthy lifestyles "age a woman's skin by 10 years." *The Telegraph*, June 4. www.telegraph.co.uk/health/healthnews/10097752/Unhealthy-lifestyles-age-a-womans-skin-by-10-years.html.

Tsindos, Spero. 2012. What drove us to drink 2 litres of water a day? *Aust N Z J Public Health* 36:207.

Turati, F. et al. 2013. Efficacy of cosmetic products in cellulite reduction: Systematic review and meta-analysis. *J Eur Acad Dermatol Venereol* 28:1. This is a terrific review of available evidence.

Valenti, D.M. et al. 2012. Effect of topical clay application on the synthesis of collagen in skin: An experimental study. *Clin Exp Dermatol* 37:164. This is one of the few studies on the potential benefits of facials on skin. It is a small animal study.

Wakefield, Melanie et al. 2003. Role of the media in influencing trajectories of youth smoking. *Addiction* 98:79. This is an excellent review of the complex role of media on smoking behavior, noting, inter alia, that "the media act as a source of observational learning by providing models which teenagers may seek to emulate."

Ward, Sarah. 2008. Spa industry worth $255 billion. *European Spa*. www.raisondetrespas.com/wp-content/uploads/2012/02/Global-Spa-business-2008.pdf.

Wolf, R. et al. 2010. Nutrition and water: Drinking eight glasses of water a day ensures proper skin hydration—myth or reality? *Clin Dermatol* 28:380.

World Health Organization. n.d. Tobacco. www.who.int/mediacentre/factsheets/fs339/en/. This offers statistics on health risks associated with smoking.

———. n.d. The truth about a suntan. www.who.int/uv/faq/uvhealtfac/en/index2.html. This is a nice summary of the impact of UV light, including an emphasis on the fact that "there is no such thing as a healthy tan!"

Wright, Brittany, Annaliese Simm and Robert McMillen. Smoking initiation and exposure to actors using tobacco. *Mississippi Tobacco Data*. http://surveillance.mstobaccodata.org/wp-content/uploads/2010/06/smoking-initiation-actors.pdf.

CHAPTER 3: PAMELA ANDERSON'S BREASTS

AFP Relaxnews. 2013. Double-jaw surgery is the latest extreme addition to South Korea's plastic surgery fad. *Daily News*, May 28. www.nydailynews .com/life-style/health/s-korea-painful-beauty-fad-bone-cutting-jaw -surgery-article-1.1356287.

American Academy of Facial Plastic and Reconstructive Surgery. 2013. Annual AAFPRS survey finds "selfie" trend increases demand for facial plastic surgery influence on elective surgery. AAFPRS, March. www .aafprs.org/media/stats_polls/m_stats.html.

American Society of Plastic Surgeons. 2012. 2012 Plastic Surgery Statistics Report. www.plasticsurgery.org/Documents/news-resources/ statistics/2012-Plastic-Surgery-Statistics/full-plastic-surgery-statistics- report.pdf.

American Society for Aesthetic Plastic Surgery. 2013. Rising demand for female cosmetic genital surgery begets new beautification techniques. *PRWeb*, April 15. www.prweb.com/releases/plastic-surgery/04/prweb 10614540.htm. This includes statistics on the number of cosmetic vagina surgeries.

Braun, Virginia. 2010. Female genital cosmetic surgery: A critical review of current knowledge and contemporary debates. *J Womens Health* 19:1393. Braun writes: "The article demonstrates a paucity of scientific knowledge and highlights a pressing need to consider the broader ramifications of surgical practices."

Burton, Laini. 2012. Nobody's fool: Power and agency in performing "The Blonde." *Critical Studies in Fashion and Beauty* 3:131–40. This article explores how various celebrities have appropriated the blonde stereotype as "a deliberate move to occupy a powerful visible space."

Carpenter, Susan. 2012. Plastic surgery—it's a guy thing too. *Los Angeles Times*, April 15. http://articles.latimes.com/2012/apr/15/image/la-ig -male-plastic-surgery-20120415.

Chae, Jiyoung. 2011. "Yes! I Had Cosmetic Surgery": Celebrities' cosmetic surgery confessions in the media and their impact on Korean female college students' perceptions. *2010 Proceedings of the New York State Communication Association* 2010: article 4.

Chauhan, Nitin et al. 2012. Perceived age change after aesthetic facial surgical procedures. *Arch Facial Plast Surg* 14:258.

Dixon, Hayley. 2013. Don't promise women they will be more beautiful, cosmetic surgeons warned. *The Telegraph*, January 29. www.telegraph .co.uk/health/healthnews/9833321/Dont-promise-women-they-will-be -more-beautiful-cosmetic-surgeons-warned.html. This article is on the Royal College report that contains the quote from Rumsey.

The Economist Online. 2012. A cut above. *The Economist*, April 23. www .economist.com/blogs/graphicdetail/2012/04/daily-chart-13.Korea ranks as the country where the most plastic surgery is performed.

FDA. n.d. Breast implants. www.fda.gov/MedicalDevices/Productsand MedicalProcedures/ImplantsandProsthetics/BreastImplants/default.htm.

Fogel, Curtis A., and Andrea Quinlan. 2011. Lady Gaga and feminism: A critical debate. *Cross-cultural Communication* 7:184–88. This is an example of an academic article questioning the degree to which performers like Lady Gaga forward a feminist agenda, "generating unrealistic expectations of female empowerment."

Griffith, James et al. 2013. Pornography actresses: An assessment of the damaged goods hypothesis. *The Journal of Sex Research* 50:621–32. This is one of the few studies to explore the attitudes of porn stars, including why they are attracted to the industry. It is also worth noting that the study found that porn stars had higher levels of self-esteem and positive feelings than the average woman. They were, however, more likely to have tried a variety of drugs—an issue noted by the actors I interviewed.

Hamermesh, Daniel, and Jeff Biddle. 1994. Looks and the labour market. *Am Econ Rev* 84:1174. This is one of Hamermesh's well-known studies on income and looks.

Hamermesh, Daniel S., and Jason Abrevaya. 2013. Beauty is the promise of happiness. *Eur Econ Rev* 64:351. This is an international study on the direct and indirect impact of beauty on happiness.

Hamermesh, Daniel S., Xin Meng and Junsen Zhang. 2002. Dress for success: Does primping pay? *Labour Econ* 9:361.

Han, Seunghwa Madeleine. 2012. Pretty in plastic: K-Pop and Korea's plastic surgery boom. *New America Media*, December 30. http://

newamericamedia.org/2012/12/pretty-in-plastic----k-pop-and-koreas-plastic-surgery-boom.php. This includes the quote on the percentage of teenagers getting plastic surgery and the desire to look like a K-Pop star.

The Harris Poll. 2012. One in five U.S. adults now has a tattoo. *Harris Interactive*, February 23. www.harrisinteractive.com/NewsRoom/Harris Polls/tabid/447/mid/1508/articleId/970/ctl/ReadCustom%20Default/Default.aspx.

Holliday, Ruth, and Joanna Elfving-Hwang. 2012. Gender, globalization and aesthetic surgery in South Korea. *Body & Society* 18:58. This is a nice analysis of the plastic surgery phenomenon in South Korea.

Imadojemu, Sotonye et al. 2013. Influence of surgical and minimally invasive facial cosmetic procedures on psychosocial outcomes: A systematic review. *JAMA Dermatol* 149:1325–33.

International Society of Aesthetic Surgery. 2008. Celebrity influences on plastic surgery. www.isaps.org/. This survey ranked Pamela Anderson as the person with the most sought-after breasts.

Jones, Barry, and Steven J. Lo. 2012. How long does a face lift last? Objective and subjective measurements over a 5-year period. *Plast Reconstr Surg* 130: 1317.

Karimi, Kian et al. 2011. The efficacy of rhinoplasty alone in facial rejuvenation. *Am J Otolaryngol* 32:269. The finding was that nose jobs alone were not rejuvenating.

Kelly, B., and C. Foster. 2012. Should female genital cosmetic surgery and genital piercing be regarded ethically and legally as female genital mutilation? *BJOG* 119: 389. This paper argues that genital cosmetic surgery should not be legal.

Kosut, Mary. 2006. An ironic fad: The commodification and consumption of tattoos. *J Pop Cult* 39:1035.

Lee, Soohyung, and Keunkwan Ryu. 2012. Plastic surgery: Investment in human capital or consumption? *J Hum Cap* 6:224. This study concludes that cosmetic surgery does not improve looks sufficiently to make it worthwhile from an economic perspective.

Liao, Lih-Mei, and Sarah M. Creighton. 2011. Female genital cosmetic surgery: A new dilemma for GPs. *Br J Gen Pract* 61:7. This review article notes the risks and ethical issues associated with "designer vaginas."

Liao, Lih-Mei, et al. 2012. An analysis of the content and clinical implications of online advertisements for female genital cosmetic surgery. *BMJ Open* 2 (6). This is a study of the advertising for vagina surgery.

Maltby, J., and L. Day. 2011. Celebrity worship and incidence of elective cosmetic surgery: Evidence of a link among young adults. *J Adolesc Health* 49:483.

Margráf, J., A.H. Meyer and K.L. Lavallee. 2013. Well-being from the knife? Psychological effects of aesthetic surgery. *Clin Psychol Sci* 1:239. This study found most people were happy with the results of cosmetic surgery.

Michala, Lina, Lih-Mei Liao and Sarah M. Creighton. 2012. Female genital cosmetic surgery: How can clinicians act in women's best interests? *The Obstetrician & Gynaecologist* 14:203. The authors write: "There is limited evidence to allow women to give informed consent."

Moran, C., and C. Lee. 2013. What's normal? Influencing women's perceptions of normal genitalia: An experiment involving exposure to modified and nonmodified images. *BJOG: An International Journal of Obstetrics & Gynaecology* 121 (6): 761–66.

Pappas, Stephanie. 2013. The porn myth: Uncovering the truth about sex stars. LiveScience, February 25. www.livescience.com/27428-truth-about-porn-stars.html. This is a report on the myths surrounding porn stars.

Quoidbach, Jordi et al. 2013. The end of history illusion. *Science* 339:96. This study explores how poor we are at predicting how much we change over time.

Roxbury, Christopher et al. 2012. Impact of crooked nose rhinoplasty on observer perceptions of attractiveness. *Laryngoscope* 122:773. This offers an example of cosmetic surgery improving attractiveness by correcting an anomaly.

Royal College of Obstetricians and Gynaecologists. 2009. Study raises concerns about cosmetic labial surgery. Royal College of Obstetricians and Gynaecologists, November 11. www.rcog.org.uk/news/bjog-release-study-raises-concerns-about-cosmetic-labial-surgery.

REFERENCES AND NOTES

Ruffle, Bradley, and Ze'ev Shtudiner. 2010. Are good-looking people more employable? *Management Science,* Discussion Paper No. 10-06. This study includes data on good looks and employability, a big advantage for men but not for women. The authors speculate that "female jealousy of attractive women in the workplace is a primary reason for the punishment of attractive women."

Sarwer, David B. et al. 2002. An investigation of changes in body image following cosmetic surgery. *Plastic and Reconstructive Surgery* 109:363. This is a study on the impact of plastic surgery on overall body image and happiness.

Sarwer, David B. et al. 2008. Two-year results of a prospective, multi-site investigation of patient satisfaction and psychosocial status following cosmetic surgery. *Aesthet Surg J* 28:245.

Slevec, Julie, and Marika Tiggemann. 2010. Attitudes toward cosmetic surgery in middle-aged women: Body image, aging anxiety, and the media. *Psychol Women* 34:Q 65. The authors write that the "effects of media on cosmetic surgery attitudes were primarily direct."

Sperry, Steffanie et al. 2009. Cosmetic surgery reality TV viewership. *Ann Plast Surg* 62:7. This study looked at the impact of shows like *Extreme Makeover*.

Subramanian, Courtney. 2013. Plastic surgeons say women want arms like Michelle Obama's. *Time,* April 30. http://newsfeed.time.com/2013/04/30/plastic-surgeons-say-women-want-arms-like-michelle-obamas/.

Surgical Practice Working Party. 2013. *Professional Standards for Cosmetic Practice Cosmetic.* The Royal College of Surgeons. www.rcseng.ac.uk/publications/docs/professional-standards-for-cosmetic-practice/.

Swami, Viren, Rosanne Taylor and Christine Carvalho. 2009. Acceptance of cosmetic surgery and celebrity worship: Evidence of associations among female undergraduates. *Pers Individ Dif* 47:869.

Tantleff-Dunn, Stacey. 2001. Breast and chest size: Ideals and stereotypes through the 1990s. *Sex Roles* 45:231. This article notes the role of Pamela Anderson.

United Nations. 2008. *Eliminating female genital mutilation: An interagency statement.* United Nations. www.un.org/womenwatch/daw/csw/csw52/

statements_missions/Interagency_Statement_on_Eliminating_FGM
.pdf. This statement defines the practice and calls for policy action.

Young, Katy. 2013. Michelle Obama inspires a 4000 per cent rise in upper
arm surgery. *Telegraph*, May 2. http://fashion.telegraph.co.uk/article/
TMG10031006/Michelle-Obama-inspires-a-4000-per-cent-rise-in
-upper-arm-surgery.html. This story is an example of the growing popularity of this particular cosmetic surgery. It also includes the number and
kinds of common surgeries (see also http://newsfeed.time.com/2013/04/
30/plastic-surgeons-say-women-want-arms-like-michelle-obamas/).

Zimm, A. Joshua et al. 2013. Objective assessment of perceived age reversal
and improvement in attractiveness after aging face. *JAMA Facial Plast
Surg* 15:405. This study found little improvement in appearance of age as
a result of cosmetic surgery.

CHAPTER 4: WIRED BEHAVIOR

Belot, Michèle, V. Bhaskar and Jeroen van de Ven. 2012. Beauty and the
sources of discrimination. *J Human Resources* 47 (Summer): 851. This is
a TV game show study.

Bishop, Katrina. 2013. Abercrombie hiring of hot staff challenged in Europe.
CNBC, July 29. www.cnbc.com/id/100921082.

Borland, Jeff, and Andrew Leigh. 2012. Unpacking the beauty premium:
What channels does it operate through, and has it changed over
time? *Economic Record* 90:17–32. www.scribd.com/doc/119151973/
Australian-Beauty-Borland-and-Leigh.

Buchanan, Kyle. 2013. Leading men age, but their love interests don't.
Vulture, April 18. www.vulture.com/2013/04/leading-men-age-but
-their-love-interests-dont.html. This provides a terrific breakdown on the
age gap between famous male and female onscreen couples.

Buote, Vanessa M. et al. 2011. Setting the bar: Divergent sociocultural
norms for women's and men's ideal appearance in real-world contexts.
Body Image 8:322.

Castillo, M. 2013. The benefits of beauty. *AJNR Am J Neuroradiol* 34:1. This
is a nice review of the data on the value and benefits of beauty.

Cattarin, Jill A. et al. 2000. Body image, mood, and televised images of attractiveness: The role of social comparison. *J Soc Clin Psychol* 19:220.

Etcoff, Nancy. 1999. *Survival of the prettiest.* New York: Anchor Books.

Etcoff, N.L. et al. 2011. Cosmetics as a feature of the extended human phenotype: Modulation of the perception of biologically important facial signals. *PLoS ONE* 6:e25656.

Expósito, Francisca, Inmaculada Valor-Segura and Antonio Herrera. 2012. Is miss sympathy a credible defendant alleging intimate partner violence in a trial for murder? *European Journal of Psychology Applied to Legal Context* 4:179.

Fink, Bernhard et al. 2008. Visual attention to variation in female facial skin color distribution. *J CosmetDermatol* 7:155. This study tracked what men and women look at and judge to be attractive.

Fletcher, Jason M. 2009. Beauty vs. brains: Early labor market outcomes of high school graduates. *Econ Lett* 105:321. This study showed that good-looking high school students do better than average and that there is a 3 to 5 percent "plainness penalty."

Hamblin, James. 2013. You can be too beautiful. *The Atlantic*, February 20. www.theatlantic.com/magazine/archive/2013/03/you-can-be-too-beautiful/309227/. This is a nice popular-press summary of a few of the downsides of beauty.

Johnston, David W. 2010. Physical appearance and wages: Do blondes have more fun? *Econ Lett* 108:10. This study found that blondes make more money and marry wealthier men and discusses other studies regarding social value of blond hair.

Kedia, G. et al. 2013. The neural correlates of beauty comparison. *Soc Cogn Affect Neurosci* 9:681–8.

Kenrick, Douglas T., and Sara E. Gutierres. 1980. Contrast effects and judgments of physical attractiveness: When beauty becomes a social problem. *J Pers Soc Psychol* 38:131.

———. 1989. Influence of popular erotica on judgments of strangers and mates. *J Exp Soc Psychol* 25:159.

Kushnick, Geoff. 2013. Why do the karobatak prefer women with big feet?

Flexible mate preferences and the notion that one size fits all. *Hum Nat* 24:268.

Kwart, D.G., T. Foulsham and A. Kingstone. 2012. Age and beauty are in the eye of the beholder. *Perception* 41:925. This is an example of a study that found a close link between perceptions of age and beauty.

Lauzen, Martha M., and David M. Dozier. 2005. Maintaining the double standard: Portrayals of age and gender in popular films. *Sex Roles* 52:437.

Lincoln, Anne E., and Michael Patrick Allen. 2004. Double jeopardy in Hollywood: Age and gender in the careers of film actors, 1926–1999. *Sociol Forum* 19:611.

Matts, Paul J., and Bernhard Fink. 2010. Chronic sun damage and the perception of age, health and attractiveness. *Photochem Photobiol Sci* 9:421. This is a review of evidence on how men perceive aging skin.

McNulty, James K. et al. 2008. Beyond initial attraction: Physical attractiveness in newlywed marriage. *J Fam Psychol* 22:135. There was no evidence found that being more attractive provided any benefits to marriage.

Mears, Ashley. 2010. Size zero high-end ethnic: Cultural production and the reproduction of culture in fashion modeling. *Poetics* 38:21.

Mobius, Markus M., and Tanya S. Rosenblat. 2006. Why beauty matters. *Am Econ Rev* 96:222.

Mocan, Naci H., and Erdal Tekin. 2006. Ugly criminals. 2048 IZA Discussion Papers, Institute for the Study of Labor (IZA). This study suggested that being "very attractive reduces a young adult's (ages 18–26) propensity for criminal activity."

Mulgrew, Kate E. et al. 2013. The effect of music video clips on adolescent boys' body image, mood, and schema activation. *J Youth Adolesc* 43:92–103.

Platz, Friedrich, and Reinhard Kopiez. 2012. When the eye listens: A meta-analysis of how audio-visual presentation enhances the appreciation of music performance. *Music Percept* 30:71. This study examined available data on the degree to which attractiveness influences our appreciation of music.

Rantala, M.J. et al. 2013. Facial attractiveness is related to women's cortisol and body fat, but not with immune responsiveness. *Biol Lett* 9:20130255.

This study suggests that levels of stress may impact attractiveness of women's face.

Rhodes, Gillian. 2006. The evolutionary psychology of facial beauty. *Annu Rev Psychol* 57:199. This is a nice review of relevant literature.

Samson, Nadine et al. 2010. Visible changes of female facial skin surface topography in relation to age and attractiveness perception. *J Cosmet Dermatol* 9:79. This study showed that even small, age-related changes to skin impact how the face is perceived by men.

Scott, Brent, and Andy Henion. 2013. "Ugly" finding: Unattractive workers suffer more. *Michigan State University Today*, June 19, http://msutoday .msu.edu/news/2013/ugly-finding-unattractive-workers-suffer-more/.

Scott, Brent, and Timothy Judge. 2013. Beauty, personality, and affect as antecedents of counterproductive work behavior receipt human performance. *Human Performance* 26:93. This study demonstrated that unattractive people are treated worse.

Smirnova, Michelle Hannah. 2012. A will to youth: The woman's anti-aging elixir. *Soc Sci Med* 75:1236. This study on the advertising of anti-aging products found that the consistent message implied that aging is a disease, etc.

Strahan, Erin J. et al. 2006. Comparing to perfection: How cultural norms for appearance affect social comparisons and self-image. *Body Image* 3:211. This study explored, among other things, how women are more likely to upward compare and to compare to unrealistic norms (e.g., models). The authors write: "Clearly, the standards of physical attractiveness set by models and celebrities are unrealistic for the average woman to strive for."

Swami, V. et al. 2010. More than just skin deep? Personality information influences men's ratings of the attractiveness of women's body sizes. *J Soc Psychol* 150:628.

Tesser, A., M. Millar and J. Moore. 1988. Some affective consequences of social comparison and reflection processes: The pain and pleasure of being close. *J Pers and Soc Psychol* 54:49. This is a classic article on social comparison.

Thornhill, Randy, Steven W. Gangestad and Randall Comer. 1995. Human female orgasm and mate fluctuating asymmetry. *Anim Behav* 50:1601. This study is on the relationship between orgasms and beauty.

Tifferet, Sigal, Ofir Gaziel and Yoav Baram. 2012. Guitar increases male Facebook attractiveness: Preliminary support for the sexual selection theory of music. *Letters on Evolutionary Behavioral Science* 3:4.

Tiggemann, Marika, and Belinda McGill. 2004. The role of social comparison in the effect of magazine advertisements on women's mood and body dissatisfaction. *J Soc Clin Psychol* 23:23. This study found that the effects of image type on mood and body dissatisfaction were mediated by the amount of social comparison reported. In other words, the more social comparison, the more it impacted mood, etc.

Tiggemann, Marika, and Janet Polivy. 2010. Upward and downward: Social comparison processing of thin, idealized media images. *Psychol Women* 34:Q 356. This is a study on the impact of social comparison and body image. The authors write: "results offer strong support to appearance social comparison as the mechanism by which idealized media images translate into body dissatisfaction for many women."

Tsukiura, Takashi, and Roberto Cabeza. 2010. Shared brain activity for aesthetic and moral judgments: Implications for the beauty-is-good stereotype. *SCAN* 6:138. This study used brain scan technology (fMRI) to show a connection between looks and perceptions of goodness.

von Bose, Caroline. 2012. Child stars vs. ugly ducklings: Does adolescent attractiveness contribute to the beauty premium? Working paper. https://webspace.utexas.edu/cv857/adolescentbeauty.pdf. This study found that "Adolescent beauty is positively and significantly correlated with adult earnings, and this effect is in addition to the premium for adult beauty."

Wapnick, Joel et al. 1997. Effects of physical attractiveness on evaluation of vocal performance. *Journal of Research in Music Education* 45:470.

———. 2009. Effects of non-musical attributes and excerpt duration on ratings of high-level piano performances. *Music Sci* 12:35. This study found that attractive musicians are, in the short term, rated more favorably, but "importance of attractiveness declines with increased musical exposure."

Wapnick, Joel, Jolan Kovacs Mazza and Alice-Ann Darrow. 1998. Effects of performer attractiveness, stage behavior, and dress on violin performance evaluation. *Journal of Research in Music Education* 46:510.

Williams, Ray B. 2012. Wired for success. *Psychology Today*, August 18. www.psychologytoday.com/blog/wired-success/201208/im-successful-because-im-beautiful-how-we-discriminate-in-favor-attractive.

Winter, Katy. 2013. Is your JOB the reason you can't get a date? Stress hormones created by high pressure careers make women less attractive. *Mail Online*, May 23. www.dailymail.co.uk/femail/article-2329083/Is-JOB-reason-date-Stress-hormones-created-high-pressure-careers-make-women-attractive.html. This is an example of a (less than constructive) media representation of a study that suggested stress may impact appearance (Rantala et al., 2013, noted above).

Woody, Robert H. 2013. Do better-looking musicians make better sounding music? *Psychology Today*, January 14. www.psychologytoday.com/blog/live-in-concert/201301/do-better-looking-musicians-make-better-sounding-music.

Yamamiya, Yuko et al. 2005. Women's exposure to thin-and-beautiful media images: Body image effects of media-ideal internalization and impact-reduction interventions. *Body Images* 2:74.

CHAPTER 5: BEAUTY AND/OR HEALTH?

American Psychological Association Task Force on the Sexualization of Girls. 2010. *Report of the APA Task Force on the Sexualization of Girls*. American Psychological Association. www.apa.org/pi/women/programs/girls/report-full.pdf.

Ata, Rheanna N., J.K. Thompson and B.J. Small. 2013. Effects of exposure to thin-ideal media images on body dissatisfaction: Testing the inclusion of a disclaimer versus warning label. *Body Image* 10:472. This study explored whether warning about the artificial nature of images changes their impact on body image.

Aubrey, Jennifer Stevens. 2010. Looking good versus feeling good: An investigation of media frames of health advice and their effects on women's body-related self-perceptions. *Sex Roles* 63:50. This study examined the impact of magazine articles on perceptions as to why we should stay healthy (i.e., for health or for beauty).

Boyce, Jessica A. et al. 2013. Positive fantasies or negative contrasts: The effect of media body ideals on restrained eaters' mood, weight satisfaction, and food intake. *Body Image* 10:535.

Brown S.A., D. Huber and A. Bergman. 2006. A perceived benefits and barriers scale for strenuous physical activity in college students. *Am J Health Promot* 2:137. This study explored why people exercise.

Chrisler, Joan C. et al. 2013. Suffering by comparison: Twitter users' reactions to the Victoria's Secret Fashion Show. *Body Image* 10:648.

Clarke, Laura Hurd. 2002. Older women's perceptions of ideal body weights: The tensions between health and appearance motivations for weight loss. *Ageing & Society* 22:751.

Crawford, Angus. 2013. Computer-generated "Sweetie" catches online predators. *BBC*, November 5. www.bbc.co.uk/news/uk-24818769.

Dixon, John B. et al. 2009. Motivation, readiness to change, and weight loss following adjustable gastric band surgery. *Obesity* 17:699. This study found that those who were motivated by appearance had better outcomes.

Dreisbach, Shaun. 2011. Shocking body-image news: 97% of women will be cruel to their bodies today. *Glamour,* February 11. www.glamour .com/health-fitness/2011/02/shocking-body-image-news-97-percent-of -women-will-be-cruel-to-their-bodies-today.

Eisenberg, Marla E. et al. 2012. Muscle-enhancing behaviors among adolescent girls and boys. *Pediatrics* 130:1019. This study of steroid use concluded that "the use of muscle-enhancing behaviors is substantially higher than has been previously reported and is cause for concern."

Ellis, Marie. 2013. US obesity rates on the rise: 113 million by 2022. *MNT*, September 3. www.medicalnewstoday.com/articles/265556.php.

Ferguson, Christopher J. 2013. In the eye of the beholder: Thin-ideal media affects some, but not most, viewers in a meta-analytic review of body dissatisfaction in women and men. *Psychol Pop Media Cult* 2:20. This is an excellent meta-analysis.

Ferguson, C.J. et al. 2013. Concurrent and prospective analyses of peer, television and social media influences on body dissatisfaction, eating disorder symptoms and life satisfaction in adolescent girls. *J Youth and Adolesc* 43:1–14.

Ferreira, Cláudia, José Pinto Gouveia and Cristiana Duarte. 2013. Drive for thinness as a women's strategy to avoid inferiority. *International Journal of Psychology and Psychological Therapy* 13:15. This study suggested that the drive to be thin is part of the built-in drive to be competitive and that it is associated with a range of negative feelings.

Glenn, Nicole M. et al. 2013. Exploring media representations of weight-loss surgery. *Qual Health Res* 23:631.

Grabe, S., M.L. Ward and J.S. Hyde. 2008. The role of the media in body image concerns among women: A meta-analysis of experimental and correlational studies. *Psychol Bull* 134:460.

Hlavenka, Jenilee A. 2005. Health related v. appearance related reasons for exercise: Which encourages people to maintain an exercise program? Community of Undergraduate Journals Online. www.clemson.edu/cujo/manuscript.php?manuscript_ID=118. This is a small study on reasons people exercise (not clear if peer reviewed).

Ingledew, David K., and David Markland. 2008. The role of motives in exercise participation. *Psychology & Health* 23:807. This is a study on the motives for why people exercise.

Kilpatrick, M. et al. 2005. College students' motivation for physical activity: Differentiating men's and women's motives for sport participation and exercise. *J Am Coll Health* 54:87.

LaRose, Jessica Gokee et al. 2013. Differences in motivations and weight loss behaviors in young adults and older adults in the National Weight Control Registry. *Obesity* 21:449.

Laware, Margaret R., and Chrisy Moutsatsos. 2013. "For Skin That's Us, Authentically Us": Celebrity, empowerment, and the allure of anti-aging advertisements. *Women's Studies in Communication* 36:189. This is a study on the anti-aging ads featuring Andie MacDowell and Diane Keaton.

Maltby, John et al. 2005. Intense-personal celebrity worship and body image: Evidence of a link among female adolescents. *Br J Health Psychol* 10:17.

Meier, Evelyn P., and James Gray. 2013. Facebook photo activity associated with body image disturbance in adolescent girls. *Cyberpsychology, Behaviour and Social Networking* 17:199–206.

Micali, Nadia et al. 2013. Incidence of eating disorders in the U.K.: Findings from the U.K. General Practice Research Database. *The Lancet* 381:s75. This notes significant increase in the incidence of "eating disorder not otherwise specified" between 2000 and 2009.

Moutsiana, Christina et al. 2013. Human development of the ability to learn from bad news. *PNAS* 110:16393–401. This study showed that teenagers respond better to positive messages.

O'Brien, Kerry et al. 2007. Reasons for wanting to lose weight: Different strokes for different folks. *Eating Behaviors* 8:132. This study was on why people diet, and one conclusion was that people who diet for the purpose of appearance are less happy.

Pankratow, M., T.R. Berry and T-L.F. McHugh. 2013. Effects of reading health and appearance exercise magazine articles on perceptions of attractiveness and reasons for exercise. *PLoS ONE* 8:e61894.

Putterman, Erin, and Wolfgang Linden. 2004. Appearance versus health: Does the reason for dieting affect dieting behavior? *J Behav Med* 27:185.

———. 2006. Cognitive dietary restraint and cortisol: Importance of pervasive concerns with appearance. *Appetite* 47:64.

Smeesters, Dirk. 2010. The effects of thin and heavy media images on overweight and underweight consumers: Social comparison processes and behavioral implications. *J Consum Res* 36:930. This was a study on how the weight of the observer impacts response to idealized media images.

Smink, Frédérique R.E. et al. 2012. Epidemiology of eating disorders: Incidence, prevalence and mortality rates. *Curr Psychiatry Rep* 14:406. The authors write: "Anorexia nervosa is relatively common among young women. While the overall incidence rate remained stable over the past decades, there has been an increase in the high risk-group of 15–19 year old girls."

Suisman, Jessica L. et al. 2012. Genetic and environmental influences on thin-ideal internalization. *Int J Eat Disord* 45:942. This study was on how genes influence how people internalize media images.

Tanner, Lindsey. 2014. Steroid use much higher among gay and bi teen boys. *AP,* February 3. This news report was on a study published in *Pediatrics.* The study authors speculate on the desire for an ideal physique.

Teixeira, Pedro J. et al. 2012. Exercise, physical activity, and self-determination theory: A systematic review. *Int J Behav Nutr Phys Act* 9:78. This is a terrific review of the literature.

Teixeira, Pedro J. et al. 2012. Motivation, self-determination, and long-term weight control. *Int J Behav Nutr Phys Act* 9:1.

Vartanian, Lenny R. et al. 2012. Appearance vs. health motives for exercise and for weight loss. *Psychol Sport Exerc* 13:251–56.

Wharton, C.M., T. Adams and J.S. Hampl. 2008. Weight loss practices and body weight perceptions among U.S. college students. *J Am Coll Health* 56:579.

Whitehead, Ross D. et al. 2012. Appealing to vanity: Could potential appearance improvement motivate fruit and vegetable consumption? *Am J Public Health* 102:207. This is a commentary on the use of vanity as a public health tool and a review of relevant studies.

Willis, Laura E. and Silvia Knobloch-Westerwick. 2013. Weighing women down: Messages on weight loss and body shaping in editorial content in popular women's health and fitness magazines. *Health Commun* 29:323–31. This is a study of over 5000 pages of women's magazines.

Young, Ariana F. et al. 2012. The skinny on celebrities: Parasocial relationships moderate the effects of thin media figures on women's body image. *Soc Psychol Personal Sci* 3:659. This interesting study showed that a parasocial relationship with a celebrity might reduce the negative impact of celebrity images, thus highlighting the complexity of the phenomenon.

PART II: THE ILLUSION THAT YOU TOO CAN BE A CELEBRITY

CHAPTER 6: DREAMS OF FAME AND FORTUNE

Bishop, Emily et al. 2011. Celebrity and performance in the hopes of children. *Enfance et Cultures.* www.enfanceetcultures.culture.gouv.fr/. This Australian study involved interviews with primary school kids.

Halpern, Jake. n.d. *The Fame Survey*. www.jakehalpern.com/famesurvey.php. This is a summary of a survey that included questions about being a celebrity assistant and how celebrity status was attained.

Johnson, Andrew, and Andy McSmith. 2006. Children say being famous is best thing in world. *The Independent*, December 18. www.independent .co.uk/news/uk/this-britain/children-say-being-famous-is-best-thing-in -world-429000.html. This was a news report about a study highlighting the degree to which children value fame.

JWT. 2012. The American dream in the balance. *J Walter Thompson Canada*, September 21. www.jwtcanada.ca/theamericandreaminthebalance. This marketing report notes that Americans increasingly view fame as part of the American Dream.

Kintrea, K., R. St. Clair and M. Houston. 2011. The influence of parents, places and poverty on educational attitudes and aspirations. *Joseph Rowntree Foundation*, October. www.jrf.org.uk/sites/files/jrf/ young-people-education-attitudes-full.pdf. This is one of the few studies I could locate that found that young people's aspirations are not necessarily unrealistic. At the age of 13 many had idealistic occupations drawn from sport or celebrity but this view had waned by the age of 15.

Lockwood, Penelope, and Ziva Kunda. 1997. Superstars and me: Predicting the impact of role models on the self. *J Pers and Soc Psychol* 73:91. This study found some "role models" can be discouraging, particularly if the relevant achievement seems unattainable.

News. 2009. Children would rather become popstars than teachers or lawyers. *The Telegraph*, October 1. www.telegraph.co.uk/education/ educationnews/6250626/Children-would-rather-become-popstars-than -teachers-or-lawyers.html.

CHAPTER 7: SO YOU WANT TO BE A STAR?

Avalon, Moses. 2011. What are the Vegas odds of success on today's major label record deal? *Moses Avalon*, June 29. www.mosesavalon.com/ what-are-the-vegas-odds-of-success-on-todays-major-label-record-deal/.

The BizParentz Foundation. www.bizparentz.org/home.html. This foundation provides statistics on child actors and "is a non-profit corporation providing education, advocacy, and charitable support to parents and children engaged in the entertainment industry." One location where the 20,000+ child actors stat can be found is: www.bizparentz.org/the bizness/pilotseason.html.

Book of Odds. n.d. Things likelier than being a movie star. Book of Odds. http://bookofodds.com/Daily-Life-Activities/Entertainment-Media/ Articles/A0629-Things-Likelier-Than-Being-a-Movie-Star. See also http://usnews.nbcnews.com/_news/2012/11/28/15510840-11-things -more-likely-to-happen-than-winning-the-powerball-jackpot?lite. The article lists the chance of becoming a movie star as 1 in 1.5 million. You are more likely to die in a plane crash.

Cord, Jefferson. 2010. The music industry's funny money. *The Root*, July 6. www.theroot.com/articles/culture/2010/07/the_root_investigates_who _really_gets_paid_in_the_music_industry.html. This article breaks down how much artists make for album sales and refers to the 2 percent.

Frank, Scott. 2012. How many actors are in L.A.?: An anthropologist eyes the entertainment industry. *Hollywood Sapien*, July 5. http:// hollywoodsapien.wordpress.com/about/. This article estimates that there are approximately 108,000 actors in L.A.

———. 2012. How many actors are in New York?: An anthropologist eyes the entertainment industry. *Hollywood Sapien*, December 13. http:// hollywoodsapien.wordpress.com/about/. The article estimates that there are 28,963 professional actors in NYC.

Haynes, Bryden. 2011. What are the odds of succeeding without a record deal?" *Music Think Tank*, June 22. www.musicthinktank.com/blog/ what-are-the-odds-of-succeeding-without-a-record-deal.html. This paper estimates the number of musicians in the UK who are "successful" without a record deal.

JJA Editor. 2012. Average income, jazz musicians: $23,000? *Jazz Journalists*, February 17. http://news.jazzjournalists.org/2012/02/ average-income-jazz-musicians-23000/.

Krueger, Alan B. 2013. Land of hope and dreams: Rock and roll, economics, and rebuilding the middle class. White House, June 12. www. whitehouse.gov/sites/default/files/docs/hope_and_dreams_-_final.pdf.

This is an economic analysis of the music industry, with comments on luck.

NEA Research Bulletin. 2010. Artist unemployment rates for 2008 and 2009. *National Endowment for the Arts*. www.nea.gov/research/Notes/97 -update.pdf. The bulletin states: "Unemployment rates for actors tend to be the highest among all artist occupations."

Nordicity. 2013. *Sound analysis: An examination of the Canadian independent music industry*. Canadian Independent Music Association, February. www.nordicity.com/media/201336fjtnrdeunp.pdf.

Pincus-Roth, Zachary. 2007. The feasibility of living in Manhattan on a chorus member's salary. *Playbill*, August 31. www.playbill.com/features/ article/print/110695.html. The article estimates that 88 percent of card-holding actors are unemployed in NYC at any one time.

Plait, Phil. 2008. Death by meteorite. *Discover Magazine*, October 13. http://blogs.discovermagazine.com/badastronomy/2008/10/13/death -by-meteorite#.UUdFGKV_jao. The article provides (admittedly rough!) estimation regarding the chance of being killed by an asteroid.

Price, William J. n.d. What are the odds of becoming a professional athlete? United States Sports Academy. www.thesportdigest.com/archive/article/ what-are-odds-becoming-professional-athlete.html. The article provides statistics on the chances of making it as a professional athlete. The author looks at high school seniors for his dataset.

PRLog. 2010. Over half of young people want to be famous. *PRLog*, February 17. www.prlog.org/10536256-over-half-of-young-people-want -to-be-famous.html.

Schuker, Lauren A.E. 2003. Pretty girls. *New York Observer*, August 25. http://www.voy.com/207229/209.html. This story is about IMTA participants.

Simkins, Michael. 2009. When the going gets tough. *The Guardian*, May 9. www.guardian.co.uk/stage/2009/may/09/tips-surviving-acting-industry. This editorial highlights how tough it is to find work as an actor. Simkins writes: "The old maxim still holds true: if you can think of any other career that would give you the same sense of satisfaction or peace of mind, do that instead. You'll get little of either as an actor."

Turner, Randy. 2013. Parents who can afford it scramble to get kids into elite hockey programs. *Winnipeg Free Press*, February 2. www.winnipegfree press.com/opinion/fyi/spring-fever-189487451.html. This article quotes parents' expectations regarding making it as a player in the NHL.

Wikipedia. List of electronic music genres. Wikipedia. http://en.wikipedia. org/wiki/List_of_electronic_music_genres.

CHAPTER 8: CELEBRITY DREAMS AND COGNITIVE BIASES

Atasoy, Ozgun. 2013. You are less beautiful than you think. *Scientific American*, May 21. www.scientificamerican.com/article.cfm?id=you-are -less-beautiful-than-you-think. This article summarizes relevant data on beauty.

Brim, Orville Gibert. 2009. *Look at me!: The fame motive from childhood to death*. Ann Arbor: The University of Michigan Press. This looks at, among other things, the number of individuals seeking fame.

Brown, Jonathon D. 2012. Understanding the better than average effect: Motives (still) matter. *Pers Soc Psychol Bull* 38:209. This is a nice study and review of the literature.

Catina, P. et al. 2005. Cross-cultural analysis of positive illusions and sport performance levels in American, Croatian, and Norwegian basketball players. *Coll Antropol* 29:453. This study explored optimistic bias and the related concept of positive illusion—and its relevance to the performance and attitudes of basketball players.

Chamorro-Premuzic, T. et al. 2009. Assessing pupils' intelligence through self, parental, and teacher estimates. *Educational Psychology* 29:83.

Epley, Nicholas, and David Dunning. 2000. Feeling "holier than thou": Are self-serving assessments produced by errors in self- or social prediction? *J Pers Soc Psych* 79:861. This study showed that people think they are more selfless, kind and generous than others.

Epley, Nicholas, and Erin Whitchurch. 2008. Mirror, mirror on the wall: Enhancement in self-recognition. *PSPB* 34:1159.

Frey, Bruno S., and Beat Heggli. 1989. An ipsative theory of business behavior. *J Econ Psychol* 10:l. This study notes unrealistic optimism.

Gilovich, Thomas, Dale Griffin and Daniel Kahneman, ed., 2002. *Heuristics and biases: The psychology of intuitive judgment.* Cambridge: Cambridge University Press. This is a great collection on various cognitive biases.

Johnson, Dominic D.P., and James H. Fowler. 2011. The evolution of overconfidence. *Nature* 477:317.

Jung, Verena, Sascha L. Schmidt and Benno Torgler. 2012. Antecedents of attitudes towards risky career choices. EBS Business School Research Paper No. 12-10. Available at SSRN: http://ssrn.com/abstract=2185429 or http://dx.doi.org/10.2139/ssrn.2185429.

———. 2012. What shapes young elite athletes' perception of chances in an environment of great uncertainty? CREMA Working Paper Series 2012–14, Center for Research in Economics, Management and the Arts (CREMA). http://external-apps.qut.edu.au/business/documents/discussionPapers/2012/WP292.pdf. This study demonstrated unrealistic optimism among German soccer players. It was also a nice summary of relevant literature, and included an Adam Smith quote.

Kårstad, S.B. et al. 2013. What do parents know about their children's comprehension of emotions? Accuracy of parental estimates in a community sample of pre-schoolers. *Child Care Health Dev* 40:346–53.

Kaufman, James C., Michelle L. Evans and John Baer. 2010. The American Idol effect: Are students good judges of their creativity across domains? *Empirical Studies of the Arts* 28:3. This is an interesting study of grade four students' ability to assess their own talents.

Kunreuther, Howard, Nathan Novernsky and Daniel Kahneman. 2001. Making low probabilities useful. *J Risk Uncertain* 23:103. This study showed that people "seem unresponsive to changes in the order of magnitude of a low probability."

Lench, Heather C. et al. 2006. My child is better than average: The extension and restriction of unrealistic optimism. *J Appl Soc Psychol* 36:2963. This is an example of a study that demonstrated how parents view their kids' abilities.

Plimmer, Geoff, and Alison Schmidt. 2007. Possible selves and career transition: It's who you want to be, not what you want to do. *New*

Directions for Adult and Continuing Education 2007:61. The authors write: "Unrealistic optimism can also lead to poor decisions and misplaced effort. Optimistic self-deception is highest in early adulthood and seems to decline during the life course."

Preidt, Robert. 2013. Poll: Many Americans don't see their kids as overweight. *Medline Plus*, February 25. National Institutes of Health. www.nlm.nih .gov/medlineplus/news/fullstory_134338.html.

Reyna, Valerie F., and Charles J. Brainerd. 2008. Numeracy, ratio bias, and denominator neglect in judgments of risk and probability. *Learn Individ Differ* 18:89.

Schweizer, Karl, Alexandra Beck-Seyffer and Rainer Schneider. 1999. Cognitive bias of optimism and its influence on psychological well-being. *Psychol Rep* 84:627.

Shah, Punit. 2012. Toward a neurobiology of unrealistic optimism. *Front Psychol* 3:1. This is a nice review of the science behind optimistic bias. Punit writes: "Optimism bias is a robust phenomenon with a neuro-biological basis."

Sharot, Tali et al. 2011. How unrealistic optimism is maintained in the face of reality. *Nat Neurosci* 14:1475. This is a neuroscience study on the biological basis of optimistic bias.

Sunstein, Cass R. 2003. Probability neglect: Emotions, worst cases, and law. *Yale Law Journal* 112:61.

Svenson, O. 1981. Are we less risky and more skillful than our fellow drivers? *Acta Psychologica* 47:143. Ninety-three percent of people think that they are better drivers than average.

University of Michigan Press. 2009. Q&A with Orville Gilbert Brim, author of *Look at Me!: The Fame Motive from Childhood to Death*. University of Michigan Press. www.press.umich.edu/pdf/9780472070701_qa.pdf. In this interview, Gilbert Brim suggests that there are 20,000 "fame" slots for about 4 million fame seekers.

vanVeelen, Matthijs, and Martin A. Nowak. 2011. Evolution: Selection for positive illusions. *Nature* 477:282. This editorial refers to several of the overconfidence studies, such as the survey of high school students.

vonHippel, William, and Robert Trivers. 2011. The evolution and psychology of self-deception. *Behav Brain Sci* 34:1. This nice article summarizes evolutionary aspects of self-deception.

Weinstein, N.D. 1980. Unrealistic optimism about future life events. *J Pers Soc Psychol* 39:806. This is one of the best-known papers exploring the phenomenon of unrealistic optimism.

CHAPTER 9: SIMON COWELL AND SOCIAL PRESSURE

Flack, Eric. 2012. Talent search under fire for use of Disney name. *Wave 3 News*, June 5. www.wave3.com/story/18708180/talent-search-uses -disney-name-not-really-for-disney. This is one of many stories highlighting acting scams aimed at kids.

Joseph, Marvin. 2013. Kids try on model behavior. *Washington Post*, April 5. High Beam. www.highbeam.com/doc/1P2-34482273.html.

Uhls, Y.T., and P.M. Greenfield. 2011. The value of fame: Preadolescent perceptions of popular media and their relationship to future aspirations. *Dev Psychol* 48:315. This study noted the degree to which fame is a dominant value and goal.

CHAPTER 10: LUCK, "IT" AND TEN THOUSAND HOURS

BBC News Online. 2008. Celebrity culture "harms pupils." *BBC*, March 14. http://news.bbc.co.uk/1/hi/education/7296306.stm. This story reports on UK teachers' perspectives on students' desire for fame.

Berri, D., and R. Simmons. 2009. Catching a draft: On the process of selecting quarterbacks in the National Football League amateur draft. *J Prod Anal* 35:37.

Berri, David J., and Brian Burke. 2012. Measuring productivity of NFL players. In *The Economics of the National Football League Sports*, Kevin G. Quinn, ed., Chapter 8. New York: Springer. Also published in *Economics, Management and Policy* 2:137. This paper emphasizes the challenges and complexities associated with measuring productivity.

CBC News. 2010. Interview: Paul McCartney heads to Canada. *CBC News*, August 6. www.cbc.ca/news/arts/interview-paul-mccartney-heads-to

-canada-1.942764. The interview contains McCartney's comments on the 10,000 hours theory.

Ford, Liz. 2005. Staging post. *The Guardian*, May 23. www.theguardian .com/education/2004/aug/23/choosingadegree. This reports on studies that have shown that formal training increases your chances of becoming a working actor, but chances are still slim!

Hambrick, David et al. 2013. Deliberate practice: Is that all it takes to become an expert? *Intelligence* 45:34–45.

Hamilton, Anita. 2013. It's getting harder to make money on YouTube. *Business Week*, April 22. www.businessweek.com/articles/2013-04-22/its-getting -harder-to-make-money-on-youtube. This article outlines the economics behind YouTube and notes how difficult it can be to make money there.

Kane, Brian. 2010. Balancing anonymity, popularity and micro-celebrity. *Alb L J Sci & Tech* 20:327.

Kool, Wouter, Sarah J. Getz and Matthew M. Botvinick. 2013. Neural representation of reward probability: Evidence from the illusion of control. *J Cog Neurosci* 25:852. This study mapped brain activity and the illusion of control.

Koz, D., J. Fraser-Thomas and J. Baker. 2012. Accuracy of professional sports drafts in predicting career potential. *Scand J Med Sci Sports* 22:e64. This study "highlight[ed] the challenges of accurately evaluating amateur talent."

Marsden, Sam. 2013. *The Cuckoo's Calling*: Publishers' embarrassment at turning down J.K. Rowling detective novel. *The Telegraph*, July 14. www.telegraph.co.uk/culture/books/10178960/The-Cuckoos-Calling -publishers-embarrassment-at-turning-down-JK-Rowling-detective -novel.html. This included the quote about the novel not standing out and suggesting it sold only 449 copies.

Matute, H. et al. 2007. Illusion of control in Internet users and college students. *Cyberpsychol Behav* 10:176. This is a discussion of the illusion of control.

Salganik, Matthew, and Duncan Watts. 2008. Leading the herd astray: An experimental study of self-fulfilling prophecies in an artificial cultural market. *Soc Psychol* 71:Q338. This study showed the randomness of getting a hit song. It was also mentioned in Krueger, above.

Szalavitz, Maia. 2013. 10,000 hours may not make a master after all. *Time*, May 20. http://healthland.time.com/2013/05/20/10000-hours-may -not-make-a-master-after-all/. This reviews the nature versus nurture debate in the development of greatness and expertise.

Tucker, Ross, and Malcolm Collins. 2012. What makes champions? A review of the relative contribution of genes and training to sporting success. *Br J Sports Med* 46:555.

Watts, Duncan J. 2013. J.K. Rowling and the chamber of literary fame. *Bloomberg*, July 19. www.bloomberg.com/news/2013-07-19/j-k-rowling -and-the-chamber-of-literary-fame.html.

Willis, Jonathan. 2011. The value of an NHL draft pick. *The Leafs Nation*, March 10. http://theleafsnation.com/2011/3/10/the-value-of-an-nhl -draft-pick. This is a nice summary of a few different looks at the value of draft picks. Bottom line: The first few picks are valuable and many in the first round may turn out to be "decent" players, but after that it is all fairly random.

PART III: THE ILLUSION THAT CELEBRITY STATUS IS WORTH HAVING

CHAPTER 11: A LONELY, HEALTH-DESTROYING GRIND?

Bao, Katherine Marie Jacobs. 2013. Aspirations and well-being: When are high aspirations harmful? PhD diss., University of California. www .escholarship.org/uc/item/2mb048s.

Beike, D.R., K.D. Markman and F. Karadogan. 2008. What we regret most are lost opportunities: A theory of regret intensity. *Pers Soc Psychol Bull* 35:385.

Bellis, Mark A. et al. 2007. Elvis to Eminem: Quantifying the price of fame through early mortality of European and North American rock and pop stars. *J Epidemiol Community Health* 61:896. This study found that fame increased mortality risk by more than 1.7 times.

———. 2012. Dying to be famous: Retrospective cohort study of rock and pop star mortality and its association with adverse childhood experiences. *BMJ Open* 2:e002089.

Bishop, Greg. 2009. Taking vows in a league blindsided by divorce. *NY Times*, August 8. www.nytimes.com/2009/08/09/sports/football/09marriage .html?_r=0. This article quotes statistics on the divorce rates for professional athletes.

Brickman, Philip, Dan Coates and Ronnie Janoff-Bulman. 1978. Lottery winners and accident victims: Is happiness relative? *J Pers and Soc Psychol* 36:917.

Brummelman, E. et al. 2013. My child redeems my broken dreams: On parents transferring their unfulfilled ambitions onto their child. *PLoS ONE* 8:e65360.

Click, Melissa A. et al. 2013. Making monsters: Lady Gaga, fan identification, and social media. *Popular Music and Society* 36:360–79.

Connor, J., J. Woolf and J. Mazanov. 2012. Would they dope? Revisiting the Goldman dilemma. *Br J Sports Med* 47:697. This was a study on the number of people in the general population who would take performance-enhancing drugs even if it shortened their life.

DNA India. 2009. Pattinson says best thing about being famous is staying in luxury hotels. *DNA India*, November 27. www.dnaindia.com/ entertainment/report-pattinson-says-best-thing-about-being-famous-is -staying-in-luxury-hotels-1317257. This is a quote about the few benefits of fame.

Efrat, Rafael. 2006. Bankruptcy stigma: Plausible causes for shifting norms. *Emory Bankr Dev J* 22:481.

Epstein, C.R., and R.J. Epstein. 2013. Death in *The New York Times*: The price of fame is a faster flame. *QJM* 106:517.

Gilbert, Daniel. 2006. *Stumbling on Happiness*. New York: Random House.

Gilchrist, Todd. 2012. Woody Allen on the perks of being a celebrity: "The bad stuff is greatly outweighed by the dinner reservations." *The Hollywood Reporter*, June 16. www.hollywoodreporter.com/news/woody -allen-perks-fame-rome-love-dinner-reservations-338482.

Gountas, John. 2012. Desire for fame: Scale development and association with personal goals and aspirations. *Psychology and Marketing* 29:680.

Greenberg, Jeff et al. 2010. Toward understanding the fame game: The effect of mortality salience on the appeal of fame. *Self Identity* 9:1. This study found one reason people desire fame and celebrity status is for the purpose of symbolic immortality.

Greenwood, Dara et al. 2013. Fame and the social self: The need to belong, narcissism, and relatedness predict the appeal of fame. *Pers Individ Dif* 55:490.

Halberstam, Joshua. 1984. Fame. *Am Philos* 21:Q93. Halberstam writes: "Those who desire fame as a source of pleasure believe that being famous will somehow or other improve their present lives."

Han, Xu et al. 2011. The effect of winning an Oscar Award on survival: Correcting for healthy performer survivor bias with a rank preserving structural accelerated failure time model. *Ann Appl Stat* 5:746. The authors write: "There is not strong evidence that winning an Oscar increases life expectancy." The paper also provides a nice review of literature.

Harvard Medical School. 2010. Marriage and men's health. Harvard Men's Health Watch. Harvard Health Publications, (July). www.health.harvard .edu/newsletters/Harvard_Mens_Health_Watch/2010/July/marriage -and-mens-health?utm_source=mens&utm_medium=pressre lease&utm_campaign=mens0710. This provides a nice summary of the health benefits of a good marriage.

Holt-Lunstad, J., T.B. Smith and J.B. Layton. 2010. Social relationships and mortality risk: A meta-analytic review. *PLoS Med* 7:e1000316. This includes a quote on the importance of good relationships (comparable to the health risks associated with smoking, etc.).

House, James S., Karl R. Landis and Debra Umberson. 1988. Social relation-ships and health. *Science* 241:540. This is an often-referenced paper on the value of relationships to health.

Kasser, Tim. 1996. Further examining the American Dream: Differential correlates of intrinsic and extrinsic goals. *Pers Soc Psychol Bull* 22:280. This is an often-cited paper on the impact of intrinsic and extrinsic goals on well-being.

Kaufman, Seth. 2013. Suicide rate for reality contestants three times the national average. *The King of Pain*, April 1. www.thekingofpainbook .com/2013/04/01/tkop-exclusive-suicide-rate-for-reality-contestants

-three-times-the-national-average/. This is a non-scientific analysis of suicide rates among reality-TV contestants.

Koch, Katie. 2012. Right choice, but not the intuitive one: Psychologist explores common barriers to good decision-making. *Harvard Gazette*, February 17. http://news.harvard.edu/gazette/story/2012/02/right-choice -but-not-the-intuitive-one/. This story summarizes some of Gilbert's work.

Lucas, R.E. 2007. Long-term disability is associated with lasting changes in subjective wellbeing: Evidence from two nationally representative longitudinal studies. *J Pers Soc Psychol* 92:717. This is an example of a study that found there was not complete adaptation to disability. A drop in happiness was sustained.

Luhmann, Maike et al. 2012. Subjective well-being and adaptation to life events: A meta-analysis. *J Pers Soc Psychol* 102:592. This is a nice analysis of how we respond to major life events.

Lyubomirsky, Sonja. 2011. Hedonic adaptation to positive and negative experiences. In *Oxford Handbook of Stress, Health, and Coping*, Susan Folkman, ed., 200-24. Oxford: Oxford University Press. http://sonja lyubomirsky.com/wp-content/themes/sonjalyubomirsky/papers/L2011 .pdf. This offers a useful summary of relevant literature. Also, it uses the well-known Dostoyevsky quote.

Maltby, John. 2010. An interest in fame: Confirming the measurement and empirical conceptualization of fame interest. *Br J Psychol* 101:411. This is a good analysis of the dimensions of the fame interest. Also, it refers to UK surveys on interest in fame, including a BBC story.

Maltby, John et al. 2008. Implicit theories of a desire for fame. *Br J Psychol* 99:279. This paper outlines key reasons people seek fame, including "social access" and deriving meaning by comparison to others.

Marwick, Alice E. 2011. I tweet honestly, I tweet passionately: Twitter users, context collapse, and the imagined audience. *New Media & Society* 13:114–33. This is an interesting analysis of the phenomenon of micro-celebrity and notes how the "practices of 'micro-celebrity' and personal branding, are both strategic self-[commodifying]."

Niederkrotenthaler, Thomas et al. 2012. Changes in suicide rates following media reports on celebrity suicide: A meta-analysis. *J Epidemiol Community Health* 66:1037. Suicide rates increase with reports of celebrity suicides.

Palmer, Tim. 2013. Fame can kill you sooner. *ABC*, April 18. www.abc.net .au/pm/content/2013/s3740256.htm. This is an interview with Richard Epstein about the health costs of fame.

Phys.org. 2013. Desire for fame scale can help advertisers. *Phys*, January 16. http://phys.org/news/2013-01-desire-fame-scale-advertisers.html. This is an interview with Dr. John Gountas.

Respers, Lisa France. 2013. Reality TV and suicide intertwine once again. *CNN Entertainment*, October 14. www.cnn.com/2013/10/14/showbiz/ tv/reality-tv-suicide/. This news story speculates on the connection between reality TV and suicide rates.

Rockwell, D., and D.C. Giles. 2009. Being a celebrity: A phenomenology of fame. *J Phenomenological Psychol* 40:178. This is a study on the experience of being famous.

Sheldon, Kennon M. et al. 2010. Extrinsic value orientation and affective forecasting: overestimating the rewards, underestimating the costs. *J Pers* 78:149. The authors write: "It appears that some people overestimate the emotional benefits of achieving extrinsic goals, to their potential detriment."

Sheldon, K.M., and S. Lyubomirsky. 2012. The challenge of staying happier: Testing the Hedonic Adaptation Prevention model. *Pers Soc Psychol Bull* 38:670. This study explored the impact of aspiration on levels of happiness.

Stenson, Jacqueline. 2008. Kids on steroids willing to risk it all for success. *NBC News*, March 3. www.nbcnews.com/id/22984780/. This article reviews steroid statistics.

Tierney, John. 2006. From Tinseltown to Splitsville: Just do the math. *NY Times*, September 19. www.nytimes.com/2006/09/19/opinion/19tierney .html?_r=1&scp=4&sq=Garth+Sundem&st=nyt. This article reports the "formula" for predicting how long a celebrity marriage will last (not long).

Tierney, John. 2012. Refining the formula that predicts celebrity marriages' doom. *NY Times*, March 12. www.nytimes.com/2012/03/13/science/ a-refined-formula-to-predict-doom-in-celebrity-marriages.html ?pagewanted=1&_r=1&. This is an update on the divorce formula.

Torre, Pablo S. 2009. How (and why) athletes go broke. *Sports Illustrated*, March 23. http://sportsillustrated.cnn.com/vault/article/magazine/ MAG1153364/2/index.htm.

Umberson, Debra et al. 2006. You make me sick: Marital quality and health over the life course. *J Health Soc Behav* 47:1.

Wilson, Timothy D., and Daniel Gilbert. 2005. Affective forecasting: Knowing what to want. *Curr Dir in Psychol Sci* 14:131.

Wolkewitz, M. et al. 2011. Is 27 really a dangerous age for famous musicians? Retrospective cohort study. *BMJ* 343:d7799. This study concluded that fame may increase mortality risk, but that "The 27 Club" is unlikely to be a real phenomenon.

Woodward, Gord. 2013. Fame adds life to your years, but cuts years from your life. *The Loop*, April 19. www.theloop.ca/opinion/article/ -/a/2279317/Fame-adds-life-to-your-years-but-cuts-years-from -your-life. This (highly unscientific) online survey found many willing to trade years of life for fame.

Zhang, Jie et al. 2013. Psychological strains found in the suicides of 72 celeb-rities. *J Affect Disord* 149:230. This study explored the themes present in celebrity suicides. The authors used this method to explore their theory of "strain" in the context of suicide.

CONCLUSION: THE DREAM CRUSHER

Baumeister, R.F. et al. 2003. Does high self-esteem cause better performance, interpersonal success, happiness, or healthier lifestyles? *Psychological Science in the Public Interest* 4:1–44. This analysis shows that there is little connection between self-esteem and success.

Beamon, Krystal, and Patricia A. Bell. 2002. "Going Pro": The deferential effects of high aspirations for a professional sports career on African-American student athletes and White student athletes. *Race and Society* 5:179–91.

Consumer Federation of America. 2006. How Americans view personal wealth vs. how financial planners view this wealth. Consumer Federation of America and The Financial Planning Association, January. http://www.consumerfed.org/pdfs/Financial_Planners_Study011006.pdf. This survey found that people believe a lottery is a practical way to accumulate wealth.

Couldry, Nick, and Tim Markham. 2007. Celebrity culture and public connection: Bridge or chasm? *International Journal of Cultural Studies* 10:403.

Economic Mobility Project. 2012. *Pursuing the American Dream: Economic mobility across generations.* The Pew Charitable Trusts, July. www.pewtrusts.org/en/research-and-analysis/reports/0001/01/01/pursuing-the-american-dream.

Ellen, Barbara. 2013. Cameron's quip to schoolchildren in Liberia marks him out as the class dunce. *The Guardian,* February 3. www.theguardian.com/commentisfree/2013/feb/03/cameron-liberia-education-quip. This is a nice commentary noting that a poor or underfunded education system may drive celebrity dreams.

Friedman, Howard Steven. 2012. The American myth of social mobility. *Huffington Post,* July 16. www.huffingtonpost.com/howard-steven-friedman/class-mobility_b_1676931.html. This article contains the quote about America as the land of opportunity.

Goldthwait, Bobcat. 2009. Don't be afraid to quit, success is overrated. Commencement speech given at Hampshire College, Amherst, Maine. http://boingboing.net/2012/05/22/bobcat-goldthwaite-commencemen.html.

Helliwell, John et al. 2013. *World Happiness Report.* United Nations. It should be noted that there are a variety of other happiness reports: one, produced by the OECD, places Australia at the top (www.theguardian.com/business/2013/may/28/worlds-happiest-countries-oecd-australia); another, produced by the Legatum Institute (www.li.com), is called the Prosperity Index and, in 2013, placed Norway, Switzerland and Canada at the top (www.prosperity.com/#!/?aspxerrorpath=%2Frankings.aspx). I selected the United Nations ranking as it seemed the most comprehensive and focused on the concept of "happiness."

Martin, Daniel. 2012. Britain "has worst social mobility in the Western world and becomes ingrained in children as young as three." *Mail Online*, April30.www.dailymail.co.uk/news/article-2137585/Britain-worst-social-mobility-Western-world.html. For 50 percent of British children, future wealth is tied to the status of their parents, compared to only 15 percent for those children in Denmark.

OECD. 2010. A family affair: Intergenerational social mobility across OECD countries. www.oecd.org/centrodemexico/medios/44582910.pdf.

———. 2013. PISA 2012 Results. www.oecd.org/pisa/keyfindings/pisa-2012-results-overview.pdf. This ranking of education systems shows relative poor performance of the US and the UK.

Romero, Estrella et al. 2012. Life aspirations, personality traits and subjective well-being in a Spanish sample. *European Journal of Personality* 26 (1): 45–55. This study showed the well-being associated with striving for intrinsic rewards.

Sternheimer, Karen. 2014. *Celebrity culture and the American Dream*. New York: Routledge.

Tokumitsu, Miya. 2014. In the name of love. *Jacobin*, January. www.jacobinmag.com/2014/01/in-the-name-of-love/. This is a terrific essay that argues that the idea of "do what you love" can both be exploitive and fuel disrespect for actual "work." The same, I think, can be said of the reach-for-the-stars mantra.

Twenge, Jean M. 2013. The evidence for generation me and against generation we. *Emerging Adulthood* 1:11–16.

Twenge, Jean M. and Jeffrey Arnett, 2013. A back and forth about narcissism. *New York Times*, August 5. This is an interesting debate regarding data on narcissism.

Twenge, Jean M., and W. Keith Campbell. 2009. *The Narcissism Epidemic*. New York: Free Press.

Weisenthal, Joe. 2013. Here's the new ranking of top countries in reading, science, and math. *Business Insider*, December 3. www.businessinsider.com/pisa-rankings-2013-12#ixzz2q7zqdbWG. This is a report on the OECD rankings.

INDEX

TIMOTHY CAULFIELD is a Canada Research Chair in Health Law and Policy, a Professor in the Faculty of Law and the School of Public Health, and Research Director of the Health Law Institute at the University of Alberta. His interdisciplinary research on topics like stem cells, genetics, research ethics, the public representations of science, and health policy issues has allowed him to publish over 350 academic articles. He has won numerous academic and writing awards and is a Fellow of the Royal Society of Canada, the Trudeau Foundation, and the Canadian Academy of Health Sciences. He contributes frequently for the popular press and is the author of two national bestsellers: *The Cure for Everything!: Untangling the Twisted Messages about Health, Fitness and Happiness*, and *The Science of Celebrity . . . or Is Gwyneth Paltrow Wrong About Everything?* (previously published as *Is Gwyneth Paltrow Wrong About Everything?: When Celebrity Culture and Science Clash*). His most recent book is *Relax, Dammit!: A User's Guide to the Age of Anxiety*. Caulfield also has a strong social media presence and is the host and co-producer of the documentary TV series, *A User's Guide to Cheating Death*.